Performance Standards for Laboratory Personnel

William O. Umiker, M.D., director of clinical laboratories, medical director of transfusion service, and medical director of the School of Medical Technologists at St. Joseph Hospital and Health Care Center, Lancaster, Pa.

Susan M. Yohe, administrative assistant in the clinical laboratory at St. Joseph Hospital and Health Care Center, Lancaster, Pa.

Medical Economics Books
Oradell, New Jersey 07649

Library of Congress Cataloging in Publication Data

Umiker, William O.
    Performance standards for laboratory personnel.

    Includes index.
    1. Medical technologists—Rating of.   2. Performance
standards.   I. Yohe, Susan M.   II. Title.   [DNLM:
1. Allied health personnel—Standards.   2. Laboratories—
Standards.   3. Personnel management.   QY 23 U48p]
RB37.6.U44   1983   616.07'5   83-17361
ISBN 0-87489-363-1

Design by Fred Witzig

ISBN 0-87489-363-1

Medical Economics Company Inc.
Oradell, New Jersey 07649

Printed in the United States of America

*To Shirlene Baney, Linda Dimter,
Ed Eisenhower, Wendy George, Jere Hinden,
Susan Orth, Joyce Reider, Becky
Serfass-Wagner, Susan White, Linda Witmer,
and Connie Wolf, who participated in
the formulation of our first
standards of performance*

Contents

Foreword

This book could not be more timely. As prospective payment systems for hospitals sweep across the country, the laboratory management team will be pressured to justify all existing and new staff positions on the basis of competence and productivity. The authors have provided the laboratory community with the definitive tool for this difficult task. Specific position descriptions with measurable standards of performance have been the exception rather than the rule in most laboratories. We haven't had a comprehensive how-to book with referenced lab standards. Now we do.

With an easy-to-read style, the authors lead us through the rationale, into identifying tasks, and applying appropriate measurements for them. The step-by-step instructions, liberal use of examples, and excellent references are just about everything you need to know to do it yourself. I plan to use it in my own consultation and teaching assignments.

The basic premise of the text is first to describe the job and what it requires, then identify the qualifications an individual must have to meet the standards. The examples in the appendix reflect the authors' criteria; but they do not preclude, for example, the separation of medical responsibilities from administrative and technical duties, nor do they favor one credentialing agency over another. The authors stress the need for ensuring that the job is performed by the individual who can best fulfill the duties, responsibilities, and standards.

Dr. Umiker and Ms. Yohe have given us a valuable management tool that should be in every laboratory—and put to immediate use. Laboratory managers and personnel directors can use it with the reassurance that it reflects the state of the art in clinical laboratory management.

Annamarie Barros, MA, CLS, CLMgt
Director, Health Management Analysts
Management consultant and educator
Los Gatos, California

Preface

The phenomenal growth of clinical laboratories shows no signs of abating. Dynamic technology and automation push productivity ever higher and continue to expand the menu of tests offered. Small facilities now perform tests once available only at select reference laboratories.

Because of these developments and others, today's laboratory managers spend more time planning and organizing. They must direct, motivate, and control a larger and more sophisticated staff than ever before, and they work with a lab team that has a great diversity of backgrounds, qualifications, and individual goals. Add in the factors of participatory management, quality care, and cost containment, and you have the ingredients of most laboratory managers' ultimate goal—to perform high-quality, cost-effective work in a harmonious working environment. We can meet this goal only if employees know what they are expected to do and how well to do it.

And this brings us to the need for better position descriptions and performance standards. Management consultants proclaim the virtues of these standards, but the directive to develop them usually comes from top management, as part and parcel of a decision to institute a merit-pay system. Unfortunately, such directives are seldom accompanied by specific how-tos. Top brass leaves it to the first-line supervisor to blaze the trail.

That's where we come in. We've had experience in this time-consuming chore and would like to help all you performance-standard pioneers. It's a simple goal for a difficult task. We hope this book eases your way.

Publisher's Notes

Performance Standards for Laboratory Personnel, like its companion volume, *Interviewing Skills for Laboratory Supervisors,* draws on the authors' wealth of managerial and administrative experience in hospital laboratories.

William O. Umiker, M.D., has since 1960 been director of clinical laboratories, medical director of transfusion service, and medical director of the School of Medical Technologists at St. Joseph Hospital and Health Care Center, Lancaster, Pa. He is also a member of the adjunct faculty at both Millersville (Pa.) State College and Elizabethtown (Pa.) College, a laboratory inspector for the College of American Pathologists, and a blood bank inspector for the American Association of Blood Banks. Dr. Umiker has published extensively, including over 50 articles on laboratory management. His recent book, *The Effective Laboratory Supervisor* (Medical Economics Books, 1982), has received wide acclaim.

Susan M. Yohe is administrative assistant in the clinical laboratory at St. Joseph Hospital and Health Care Center, Lancaster, Pa., and formerly worked in materials management there. She is a business student at Franklin & Marshall College and, with Dr. Umiker, is the coauthor of several articles on laboratory management in *MLO (Medical Laboratory Observer).*

1

What standards of performance stand for

The average job description spells out the employee's duties and responsibilities. The above-average job description includes the percentage of time devoted to each duty. The superior job description includes standards of performance, or SPs. This complete document lets the employee know not only what to do but also how well he's expected to carry out these tasks.

Other writers have defined performance standards as quantitative or qualitative measures for judging whether results have been achieved,[1] and as a minimum level of performance above which we measure excellence and below which we measure failure.[2] We like to describe a standard of performance as a statement of expected results, behavior, or attitude.

We have also seen other terms used as synonyms for SPs. We agree with one of them — indicator — but reject another — objective — as being more appropriately applied to short-range goals. For example, an objective to set up a new blood alcohol procedure may include performance standards that say when it is to be done, how much it should cost, and what level of precision the method must provide.

How can you use SPs? Let's count the ways

Performance standards support a whole range of managerial activities, and you'll find them well worth the effort you'll have to put into devising them. Here are the ways we use SPs.

1. To provide performance feedback to employees

Workers with documented SPs always know how well they are doing. They needn't wait for their next performance appraisal or have their supervisor constantly looking over their shoulders.

2. To increase supervisors' knowledge of their employees' responsibilities

The very act of preparing standards forces a supervisor to review everyone's duties and responsibilities. This leads to needed revisions in position descriptions.

3. To facilitate new employees' indoctrination

Whoever is responsible for the orientation and training of new employees finds it much easier with a written description of the expected level of performance.[3]

4. To help introduce new methods and instruments

We are seeing new methods and instruments with increasing frequency. Technologists must know how to use them, and with what level of proficiency.

5. To supplement coaching and counseling

Employees with good SPs need less coaching. They are more likely to ask for help when they realize they are not meeting their standards.

6. To make performance reviews easier

Standards are no substitute for supervisors' judgment of employee performance. But with them, supervisors can base that judgment on solid facts, not vague impressions and irrelevant factors. One reason supervisors and employees are so leery of performance reviews is that they're often based on such subjective factors as character traits, personality, or attitudes. SPs permit more objective, less emotional appraisals.[4]

7. To provide an objective basis for promotion and merit-pay increases

The current interest in SPs was spawned by the need for better criteria for selecting employees who deserve merit increases, bonuses, or promotions. This is especially true of organizations where productivity or quality of work is difficult to evaluate.

If this is the sole use of SPs, however, they will be of limited value. In such cases, an adversarial relationship develops as employees struggle to get standards lowered. Disagreements abound, and the motivational potential that challenge provides is lost. On the other hand, it is difficult to administer a merit-pay or promotion system without SPs.

8. To provide a sound basis for firing unsatisfactory workers

By documenting specific levels of expected performance, SPs make it apparent when someone isn't performing adequately. Unionization and labor laws have done much to protect the worker from unfair hiring and firing practices; SPs help management define unsatisfactory work practices.

9. To improve morale and motivation

Managers who advocate SPs report less grumbling and greater productivity.[5] Standards provide challenges that can motivate, provided they are not set too low or too high.

Classification of SPs

There are several ways to classify performance standards. The first grouping is according to whether they are based on results, behavior, or attitude.

SPs based on expected results are the best. They specify what the employee should accomplish and are expressed in terms of quality, time, or cost. Examples appear in Table 1-1.

SPs based on behavior, which are also called controlling standards, relate to work habits and compliance with rules, regulations, policies, and procedures. They are most appropriate for repetitive or routine tasks.[6] Table 1-2 gives some examples.

SPs based on attitude are admittedly subjective, and must therefore be handled with care, both in formulating and enforcing them. Interpretation is open to criticism because of bias or discrimination. Examples are shown in Table 1-3.

SPs may also be based on several kinds of comparisons. Historical standards compare performance with previous results. An example would be: "Maintenance costs must not exceed last year's costs by more than 5 percent."

Performance may also be compared with that of other employees, as here: "Your attendance record must be equal to or better than the average of all hospital employees." In another example, performance is measured by time studies or commonly observed results: "The turnaround time for a Stat differential blood count will be no longer than 12 minutes, excluding staining time."

Finally, we may also think of standards as being positive or negative. A positive SP states what is wanted: "A stain control using known gram-negative and gram-positive organisms shall be included in each batch of smears." Negative SPs state what is not wanted: "Overtime may not exceed an average of two hours per week per employee."

Levels of performance

When setting standards, you and the employee must know what level of performance you're aiming for—minimum, average, or superior.

The minimum level is what separates satisfactory from unsatisfactory performance. Employees whose performance falls below this level can expect to lose their jobs if their work does not improve. If you use this level alone, employees won't know when their performance is superior or in the upper average ranges. This pass-fail system is thus of limited value for promotion or merit-pay increases.

Average-level standards indicate neither unsatisfactory nor superior performance, so they aren't useful for termination, promotion, or merit-pay decisions. If they are to be used at all, it should be with other levels.

Minimum and superior levels are far more difficult to formulate. The lower level sets the pass-fail point. The upper level is the cut-off point between upper-average and superior performance. For many SPs, this can be done with percentages. Meeting a standard less than 75 percent of the time is unsatisfactory, for example, but more than 95 percent of the time is superior. These are probably the best kinds of standard to set, but, as we said, it's harder to come up with them.

Three-level standards are often favored by those who don't have to prepare them. Setting measurable standards for minimum, average, and top performance is very difficult for laboratory jobs—and probably not really necessary.

Criteria for a good standard

Now let's look at some important characteristics of SPs.

It must be linked to an important and specific responsibility

It's a waste of time preparing SPs for inconsequential activities. If failure to perform a duty satisfactorily does not jeopardize an employee's tenure, it doesn't warrant an SP.[7] A standard should specify behavior or attitudes that affect results. SPs such as "demonstrate good work habits," or "have a cooperative attitude," represent commendable traits, but they lack specificity.

It must be based on expected results

Without them, nothing is achieved. An SP states how fast something must be done in terms of deadline or turnaround time, and how well it must be done in terms of precision and accuracy.

It defines constraints

A performance standard sets precise limitations of time, safety, and cost.

It is objective, observable, or measurable

It must define quality or quantity in terms of dollars, hours, number of occurrences, or product units. Here's an example: "The monthly report must be submitted by the 10th day of the following month."

Subjective standards, on the other hand, depend on the interpretation or judgment of the manager and are therefore highly biased: "The phlebotomist must be neatly groomed."

It deals with performance over which the employee has complete control

A supervisor's standard dealing with personnel costs should be expressed in hours rather than dollars. The dollar amounts depend largely on the pay increases awarded by top management. Nor should a supervisor be held accountable for a ceiling of hours worked if the workload is not under his control.

It must be necessary, not superfluous

General codes of conduct are provided in personnel, safety, and procedure manuals. These need not be repeated as SPs unless a job demands special controls. Dress codes for phlebotomists might be an example.

It is understood and agreed on by both the employee and supervisor

SPs should be as clear to an employee as par is to a golfer. Employees cannot be expected to meet standards they don't understand. A standard that isn't written down or one that is subjective can create much misunderstanding. If an employee feels that a standard is unfair, the two of you must renegotiate it.

It is realistic

Words like "always" and "never" automatically disqualify the accompanying statement as a minimal standard. No one is perfect. Employees are frustrated by standards they know they can't achieve. Equally bad are those set below what you believe to be acceptable. In such situations, subsequent disciplinary action or termination is difficult.

It is challenging

A person usually needs a challenge to give maximum effort, and a lack of challenge is a weakness of minimum SPs. On the other hand, minimum standards must be the same for employees who perform the same functions. Setting different standards for the same work invites legal or union difficulties. Provide the challenge by setting higher superior standards or new work objectives. Table 1-4 lists items to consider when you select performance standards.

Table 1-1. Standards Based on Results

Quality

Criteria:

Precision	Errors
Accuracy	Repeats
Awards	Complaints
Commendations	Incident reports
QC statistics	QC deficiencies

Examples:

- The pathologist must find fewer than 5 percent of stained smears unsatisfactory.

- Supplies must be counted and stored by the end of the shift.

- Reports must be filed in the basement storeroom in the right order.

- There must be no more than two errors per week in charge slips.

Productivity

Criteria:

Work units or time	Deadlines
Schedules	Downtime
Turnaround time	

Examples:

- Routine surgical slides must be submitted to the pathologist before 10 a.m.

- All unsatisfactory QC results must be investigated; reports must be submitted within five working days of their receipt.

- Instrument downtime must be less than that for last year.

- Turnaround time for Stat blood glucose must be no longer than 15 minutes.

Financial

Criteria:

Budget preparation

Deviations from budget

Overtime

Cost per text

Time savers

Maintenance costs

Examples:

- Overtime must be reduced by 10 percent for this year.
- The cost of supplies must increase no more than 8 percent over last year.
- Exceptions to the budget must have the department head's approval.
- Budget items or capital expenditures must be prepared before Jan. 1, personnel budget before Feb. 1, and supply budget before March 1.

Research and development

Criteria:

Suggestions accepted

Research grants obtained
  or renewed

Papers presented or published

Research projects completed

New instruments or procedures
  tested or introduced

Examples:

- The proposed new method for compatibility tests must be evaluated by Aug. 1.
- The reference values for serum lipase must be determined by July, with statistical validity approved by the QC coordinator.

Teaching and training

Criteria:

Lecture and benchwork

Indoctrination of new employees

Training employees in new methods and instruments

Examples:

- Prepare a list of exam questions pertaining to lectures and benchwork that you give. Submit it to the school director before the start of the lecture series.
- Prepare a set of student lecture notes that the director finds acceptable no later than a week before the lecture.
- Discuss instrumentation at a laboratory staff meeting within the next three months.

Self-development and new work objectives

Criteria:

Number of new objectives proposed   CE achievements

Numbers of objectives achieved

Examples:

- Earn a master's degree in medical microbiology.
- Obtain cost information by January on the programs offered.
- Submit proposal by March for financial support and reduced work hours.
- Achieve the minimal annual CE credits as established by the laboratory administration.

Table 1-2. Standards Based on Behavior

Knowledge

Criteria:

Amount of supervision
required

Consultation to physicians
and nurses

State-of-the-art knowledge

Selection of tests

Attend meetings

Patient preparation

Professional reading

Interpretation of tests

Participation in CE programs

Examples:

- Complete an evening course on assertiveness, and earn a passing grade.
- Attend at least two outside meetings a year.

Skill

Criteria:

Care of instruments

Communication

Work habits—safety,
orderliness, cleanup

Examples:

- Attend a workshop in coagulation techniques this year.
- Demonstrate competency in operating the instrument by May.
- Correctly record the acquisition number in the daily log, on the request form, and the capsule label 95 percent of the time.

Table 1-3. Standards Based on Attitude

Toward superiors

Criteria:

Attendance	Verbal support of organization's goals and policies
Participation at meetings	
Participation at social events	Conforming to dress code and other regulations
Suggestions	

Examples:

- Wear designated uniform.
- No valid complaints of bad-mouthing the department or organization outside the laboratory.
- Serve willingly on such hospital committees as recreation, and the annual hospital fair.

Toward peers

Criteria:

Participation in meetings	Coordination
Sharing	

Examples:

- Participate actively in the weekly laboratory staff meeting.
- Accept appointments to standing and ad hoc committees.
- No valid complaints concerning failure to share equipment such as centrifuges, microscopes, and refrigerator space.

Toward subordinates

Criteria:

Communication	Motivating
Delegation	Training
Coaching and counseling	Serving as mentor
Disciplining	Evaluating

Examples:

- Train a bench tech within 10 months to perform routine toxicologic analyses.

- Hold formal performance reviews at least annually.

- The lab manager must rate as satisfactory all reports of performance reviews.

- Hold a minimum of one section meeting per month.

Table 1-4. Performance Standards: Some Suggested Items

Quality

Filing errors
Complaints received
Standard deviation
Coefficient of variation and errors
Sensitivity and specificity
Proficiency reports

Productivity

Units or tests per hour
Participation in quality circles
Turnaround time
Problems overcome

Percentage of goals met
Reports completed on time
Instrument downtime

Financial

Cost control
Expenses
Number and value of new cost-containment measures
Overtime costs
Estimates compared with actual expenditures
Product selection
Inventory control

Training and education

Participation in training activities
Completion of courses
Number of training programs
Formal performance interviews held per employee
Number of educational meetings

Employee supervision

Complaints or grievances registered
Complaints received
Results of morale survey
Tardiness
Resignations
Involuntary separations
Number and quality of performance reviews
Days absent
Days sick
Number of visits to the first-aid room
Number of compensation claims
Accident frequency rate

Research and development

Research projects completed on time and within budget
Recommendations accepted and implemented
Hours spent
Ideas submitted
Papers published and submitted
Grants awarded
New procedures introduced

References

1. Allan, P., and Rosenberg, S. Formulating usable objectives for manager performance appraisal, *Personnel Journal,* Nov. 1978, p. 626.

2. Truell, G. F. *Performance Appraisal: Current Issues and New Directions,* PAT Publications. Buffalo, N.Y.

3. Umiker, W. O. Good position descriptions help fit the employee to the job, *MLO,* Sept. 1981, p. 32.

4. Umiker, W. O. SPs belong in your managerial portfolio, *MLO,* April 1981, p. 33.

5. Kyser, R. C. Jr., and Mead, J. Work measurement: America's answer to the productivity challenge, *Supervisory Management,* Oct. 1981, p. 30.

6. Pitts, R. E., and Thompson, K. The supervisor's survival guide: Using job behavior to measure employee performance, *Supervisory Management,* Jan. 1979, p. 23.

7. Alexander, J. O. Making managers accountable: Develop objective performance standards, *Management Review,* Dec. 1980, p. 43.

2

Getting started: defining duties and responsibilities

There are four steps in the development and implementation of performance standards: 1) clarify what the employee is expected to do; 2) state how well it must be done; 3) develop an action plan; and 4) follow up. We'll examine each in turn, devoting this chapter to the first one.

Clarify what the employee is expected to do

Prepare or revise the position description

Performance standards must be based on a position description that defines the qualifications for and duties of the job. Each standard is linked to a duty, so omitting a duty results in omitting its standard or standards of performance.

Strong standards can't be built on weak position descriptions. Faced with a long list of minor responsibilities, a supervisor is likely to give up in despair when attempting to formulate SPs. In such a case, it's often easier to scrap an old position description and get a fresh start.

First list the three to five major functions of the position. Rank them in order of their importance or percentage of time they take. Divide each major area of accountability into smaller segments, and assign a time factor to each. For a chemistry technologist, your worksheet may look something like the example in Table 2-1.

Since most of us think in terms of absolute time values rather than in percentages, the conversion factors in Table 2-2 are helpful in estimating these percentages. If you find that certain responsibilities merit a higher priority than what their time factors indicate, highlight them on your worksheet to remind yourself that they need some special attention.

Review the list of duties and responsibilities

Carefully assess the priority and percentage of time for each item. Don't proceed until you are satisfied with every one of them. Are there unimportant items that you can delete? Do you need more study to determine how much time an employee is using for an activity?

A pivotal decision is whether a position warrants a professional-level laboratorian, such as a medical technologist, or a lesser-trained person, such as a medical technician. The duties and responsibilities as well as the standards must reflect the professional and technical qualifications. Having certain qualifications does not in itself mean that someone is performing that level of work. If a technologist does only the work of a technician, for example, the position should be that of a technician, not a technologist.

The Civil Service Commission makes a clear distinction between the two levels in its medical technologist and medical technician series.[1] Among the duties that reflect professional-level work are the following: 1) performing newer or more complex tests; 2) engaging in research and development; 3) developing quality assurance programs or implementing quality control measures; 4) formulating instructions and procedures; 5) planning or conducting training programs; and 6) recommending new tests. Table 2-3 gives more clarification. Above all, don't start work on performance standards until you are satisfied with the position description.

List future objectives on a separate sheet

They can be short- or long-term goals. Here are some examples: setting up a new procedure, evaluating an instrument, expanding a service, establishing quality control measures, reviewing data, writing a scientific paper, or developing a new policy.

Objectives frequently relate to self-development. Employees may need additional education or training to narrow their development gaps or to prepare for transfer or promotion. Table 2-4 shows more examples of typical objectives, along with some suggested standards.

Review the employee's new performance objectives

It will help to ask yourself the following questions:

- Are they compatible with the goals of the organization, the department, and my own personal goals?
- Do they include long-term as well as short-term plans?
- Are they results oriented?
- Are they relevant, realistic, understandable, measurable, and specific?
- Do they include those aimed at narrowing the employee's development gap?
- If the employee is a supervisor, do they include activities related to his work group?

If you don't have or don't like your answers to these questions, jot down those you want to rework, those you want to discuss with the employee or someone else, and those for which you need more information.

Table 2-1. Job breakdown for chemistry technologist

Major functions	Percentage of time	
Analyze specimens	85%	
Biochemical analyzer		40%
Electrolytes		20
Stat tests		10
Electrophoresis		10
Routine urinalysis		5
Teach biochemical methodology	10	
Benchwork		8
Lectures		2
Phlebotomies	5	

Table 2-2. Time/percentage conversion table*

Percentage of time	1%	5%	10%	25%	100%
Minutes/day	5	24	48	120	480
Hours/day	—	½	1	2	8
Hours/week	½	2	4	10	40
Hours/month	2	9	18	44	176

*The figures are approximate.

Table 2-3. Comparing standards appropriate for medical technologists and for medical technicians*

For technologists

Recognizes deviations from expected results, analyzes problems on scientific principles, and modifies tests to eliminate technical problems

Is familiar with reference ranges, knows expected deviations from normal in various disease states, and interprets results within the framework of the discipline

Can explain the scientific basis for diagnostic tests to students and trainees

Contacts physicians or other professional personnel to obtain additional information relating to tests, or to discuss laboratory findings

Is familiar with sensitivity, specificity, and predictive values for various laboratory procedures or instruments

For technicians

Knows when a test does not come out right, may repeat it, reports problem to superior; is not expected to analyze causes or to alter test procedure

Is not expected to know reference ranges, standard deviations, or how to interpret results

Is expected to know only the technical steps of a laboratory procedure

Calls Stats and other reports to the floor as prescribed in procedure manuals

Does not need to know sensitivity, specificity, or predictive values

*Modified from Civil Service Commission Series.

Table 2-4. Sample performance objectives with standards

Attend at least one outside professional seminar

1. The meeting must result in at least one procedural change in the section.
2. Expenses must not exceed amount allocated by the supervisor.
3. The new information must be presented at a section meeting within two months of the seminar.

Expand the donor recruitment program

1. The program must include school visits and a donor plan follow-up.
2. The program must not exceed the recruitment budget.
3. A 5 percent increase in donors must be realized.

Present a seminar to students on test taking

1. Must incur no extra costs.
2. The session must be presented during the first quarter of the school year.
3. Students must evaluate the presentation as at least "good" on a poor-fair-good-excellent scale.

Compile a slide series for orienting prospective students

1. Cost of the slides must not exceed $500.
2. The slides and presentation must be completed by Oct. 1.

Increase hospital coverage by the blood collection team

1. Weekend shifts must be staffed with at least one phlebotomist by the end of the year.
2. Section personnel budget must not be exceeded.

3. The time that medical technologists spend on weekend blood collection must be decreased by 50 percent.

Improve quality of laboratory section meetings

1. Must incur no additional costs.

2. Section employees must rate the meetings as "good" on a poor-fair-good-excellent scale.

3. Agenda must be approved by the pathologist director.

4. Must receive fewer complaints from employees.

5. At least 75 percent of section employees must attend each meeting.

Prepare a manual on orientation of new physicians to the lab

1. Manual must be completed by the end of the year.

2. Manual must eliminate at least 30 percent of calls and questions from new physicians and their office staffs.

3. Manual must include all laboratory services.

Establish an automated or semiautomated system of identification and susceptibility procedures

1. Must not exceed microbiology supply budget.

2. Must use no more than 80 hours of additional technologist time.

3. The recommendation on a specific system must be included in next year's capital budget, thus given to the financial officer by July 31 this year.

4. The recommended system must reduce turnaround time by 24 hours or more, at no increase in test cost.

5. There must be no decrease in quality of results.

Implement a word-processing system in the laboratory office

1. All medical transcriptionists must be fully trained by the end of the year as demonstrated by their performance on the equipment and by completion of the hospital-sponsored word-processing course.

2. The training must not exceed 40 hours per transcriptionist.

3. Student notes and tests must be entered on disks by next June 30.

Obtain an SBB certification

1. Must earn the certificate by next June 30.

2. All preparation must be on the employee's own time.

Reference

1. Medical Technologist Series GS-644 and Medical Technician Series GS-645 (TS72), U.S. Civil Service Commission, Feb. 1968.

Suggested reading

Truell, G. F. *Performance Appraisal: Current issues and new directions.* PAT Publications, Buffalo, N.Y.

Alexander, J. O. *Making managers accountable: Develop objective performance standards, Management Review,* Dec. 1980, p. 43.

Levels of Practice, American Society for Medical Technology, Houston, 1982.

3

How well the work must be done

Here's the crux of the matter — setting the standards, deciding what will and will not be acceptable, and determining the levels of performance.

We like the idea of formulating objectives and standards in stages, progressing from basic to more sophisticated ones, even though the state of this art is not yet highly developed.[1] We may have to be satisfied with statements that are not as precise as we would like. Periodic modifications, dictated by experience, can make the standards of performance more practical and useful. The formulation process itself provides opportunities to define better what we expect of our employees and to sharpen our planning skills.

Gathering data

Many sources of information can help in formulating SPs. Here are some of them.

Position descriptions

As we said in Chapter 2, SPs must be based on clear, concise descriptions of duties and responsibilities. Standards are, in fact, logical extensions of stated duties. "To operate an ABC instrument daily," for example, automatically suggests criteria of precision, maintenance, and safety.

Work measurement studies

Industry uses time studies and work sampling to set reasonable but challenging productivity goals. Laboratory managers seldom have the time or the interest to undertake such investigations. Fortunately, the College of American Pathologists has done much of this work for us with its workload recording method.[2] You can use its work units as standards, especially for section supervisors. Here's an example: "The annual paid-hour productivity for the hematology section shall exceed 45."

Published data

Productivity levels for certain activities can also be based on studies reported by professional organizations or medical centers. Some examples here might be the number of cytological smears screened per day, week, or month; or the degree of precision that others have achieved using a specific instrument or method.

Another excellent source for standards is the National Committee for Clinical Laboratory Standards.[3] It publishes detailed, precise guidelines for a wide range of laboratory procedures.

Committee requirements

Hospital and medical staff committees make demands on laboratory services that can be translated into performance standards. The requirements that follow are typical:

From the transfusion committee:

- Maintain a specified minimum blood inventory;
- Have available a specified amount of Rh-negative blood for emergencies;
- Do not exceed a specified percentage of units of outdated blood.

From the infection control committee:

- Report nosocomial infections;
- Report antibiotic bacterial susceptibility patterns;
- Report communicable diseases to appropriate departments of health;
- Cooperate with the infection surveillance officer.

29

From the tissue committee:

- Flag surgical cases with normal tissues;
- Prepare lists of operative cases in which no tissue was submitted to pathologists.

From the trauma committee:

- Assure adequate hematology, immunohematology, and chemistry services on second and third shifts.

From the safety committee:

- Report laboratory-acquired injuries or infections;
- Keep such incidents to a minimum;
- Report safety violations.

Policies, regulations, and procedures

In general, it's not necessary to clutter up SPs with items that are spelled out in policy and procedure manuals. Some jobs, however, have special constraints. A rigid dress code may be more appropriate for phlebotomists than for bench technologists. Long hair is less of a problem for office workers than for technologists. Members of the early morning phlebotomy team must be on time. Errors by immunohematology technologists are least likely to be tolerated. Supervisors can find policies and regulations helpful in preparing position descriptions or reports, maintaining safety and discipline, and conforming to labor laws.

Performance records

Unless the employee is a newcomer, these document past behavior, achievements, and weaknesses.

Personal observation

Managers should know which expectations are important and realistic. They see how well other employees do the same work. Superior performers demonstrate what is possible. Incompetent workers reveal what must be avoided.

The employee

He may suggest that certain SPs should be modified. This is one of the valuable tidbits gleaned from exit interviews.

How many standards and how tough should they be?

Three or four standards for each duty is average; but some responsibilities need more, some need only one. Long lists of standards usually call for severe pruning.

As for the level of performance, if you're using only one, it is usually pegged at the breakpoint between satisfactory and unsatisfactory—a minimum level. Setting average and superior levels is also possible, as we mentioned in Chapter 1. We started with minimum levels, but when our hospital introduced a merit-pay system, we had to delineate superior performance. We thus changed to a scheme with two cutoff points. One is between satisfactory and unsatisfactory; the other, between average and superior.

For standards that can be expressed in percentages, pick a figure such as 70 percent or 75 percent as a minimum level. Designate performance above 90 percent or 95 percent as superior.

The breakpoint between average and superior performance should be tagged at a level consonant with the percentage of employees you want to designate as superior. If your organization wants to recognize the top 15 percent as top performers, for example, select a high breakpoint. But if half the staff will receive merit raises, set the discrimination point closer to average performance.

When you can't translate things into percentages, state specifically what unsatisfactory or superior performance is: "More than three transcription errors per month is unacceptable," or "One error a month or less represents superior work."

Formulating standards for routine duties

Begin with the most important duty, and list the conditions that define correct performance. Think in terms of quantity — how much must be done; quality — how accurately and with what precision; time — when and how fast; and manner — how diplomatically or enthusiastically the employee must do the job.

Picture the ideal employee performing a task. What actions or results stand out? Use that to formulate the standard. Now visualize an incompetent person struggling with the same work. Think about what is likely to go wrong. Will you get complaints from a patient or physician? A broken instrument? Contaminated reagents? Use this concept to design negative standards: "No more than 5 percent unsuccessful venipunctures are acceptable," or "There must be no bloodstains on the patients' bed clothes." For example:

Duty. Perform designated QC procedures.

Standard. There must be no more than two valid complaints per year from the supervisor. Must sign the logbooks when performing QC procedures at least 90 percent of the time.

Also consider what constraints must be observed, as here: "During slow periods, phlebotomists shall not socialize in the laboratory work area"; and what is completely unacceptable: "alcohol on the breath," or "long fingernails."

Keep thinking along these lines to sharpen your sense of what is and what isn't acceptable.

Use time criteria with caution. There is a natural tendency to tag on a time restriction for each task because it is so easy to do. Performing a task too quickly may compromise quality, however. When you introduce a time factor, it must be balanced with standards of quality. To decide whether time is important, ask yourself what happens if the time limit isn't met. Speed is important in performing a Stat test, but it doesn't make sense to demand that supervisors hand in QC reports at 4:30 p.m. if they can stay later to complete them.

Standards for new and nonroutine work objectives

For routine duties, spell out work habits, attitudes, and productivity. For nonrecurring tasks, however, schedules, cost containment, and end results are more appropriate. Here's an example:

New work objective. To evaluate the proposed new method for compatibility testing.

Standard. The QC coordinator will establish criteria. Costs for reagents will not exceed $400, and the target date for a preliminary report is next April.

SPs for objectives relating to self-development can be tricky. It's one thing to formulate simple standards such as achieving a passing grade in a college course or attending a workshop. More difficult is formulating a standard that measures practical application of such knowledge.

Major objectives such as developing a new service or opening a branch laboratory mandate a larger number of SPs. These include a time frame, cost constraints, and forecasting potential use and needs for training, space, and equipment.

Performance standards for managers

Because of managers' more wide-ranging duties, their performance standards are far more numerous. A glance at the position descriptions in Appendix A will quickly confirm this. Managers are responsible for many operational routines and sophisticated technological systems, and they must understand stringent requirements and societal forces.

Laboratory medicine is dynamic and complex, and the dollar cost is great. This is translated into many short-, intermediate-, and long-range objectives. The time span between planning and results achieved is proportionate to one's place in the organization. Results achieved by a chief executive officer are often measured in years.

It's easy to get bogged down with minutiae by listing countless picayune functions or objectives. Avoid this trap by starting with the manager's major functions, rather than a long menu of duties and responsibilities. Table 3-1 shows which duties lie within the various functions.

Review the SPs

When you have established the standards for one duty, review them before going on to the next. Keep the following questions in mind:

Are they understandable?

Does the person know exactly what is expected? Par in golf, for instance, tells a golfer how well he is doing at each hole and also at the end of the round when he totals up his score.

Does the employee have control of the activity?

This has been called the credit-blame criterion.[4] If the standard hasn't been met, is the employee entirely to blame? If accomplished, will he get all the credit?

Are they realistic and fair?

If this is a minimum standard, is it really that? Will you let employees stay on the job indefinitely if they fail to meet the standard? If so, then it is not a minimum standard.

If the SP is geared to differentiate between average and superior performance, does it? If it's too low, everyone doing that task must be rated superior. The indicator provides no challenge. If it's too high, employees will be frustrated and may lose deserved merit-pay increases or promotions.

To be fair, a standard must not demand a higher level of performance for one employee than for another doing the same work. Violations of this rule may invoke charges of discrimination. There are jobs in which individual differences in SPs *are* warranted. We already mentioned dress code and tardiness. Another example is the level of telephone courtesy expected of office personnel who talk to people outside the laboratory, as opposed to laboratory personnel who communicate only with each other.

Do they include forbidden words?

If you find certain words — *effective, efficient, suitable, satisfactory, adequate,* or *professional* — sprinkled throughout the standards, modify them precisely or replace them with more definite terms.

Such absolutes as *always, never,* and *without exception* are seldom appropriate either. They may be used, however, to forbid certain violations of rules or, of course, illegal acts — gross negligence, theft, or refusal to obey a lawful order.

Are they objective, specific, and measurable?

They should be all of these. Use percentages when possible. Though managers object on the basis that percentages are no better than guesstimates, we think they come close enough. We don't document the hits and misses, and we have yet to calculate an actual percentage. But the purpose of an SP is to give the employee a ballpark figure of what is expected.

If someone is falling below a required percentage, both of you will probably know it without any official tally. In cases of disagreement, you'll have to keep a record, but we have never found it necessary. Nor has this requirement added time to our supervisory duties.

When you have made the necessary changes, look over the list one last time to eliminate nonessentials. Some people become so enamored of this technique that they start to measure everything. This can result in a confusing array of objectives and standards that ends up requiring time-consuming observations or reporting.[4]

When you are satisfied with your SPs, flag those that someone else will evaluate. Record their names after each standard. Make certain that these people and the employee are aware of that assignment. Don't wait until the next performance review to get feedback from these observers.

A last word here. Before you undertake the preparation of SPs, check over the dos and don'ts in Table 3-2.

Table 3-1. A manager's major functions and the duties associated with them

Function	Duties
Planning	Establish a departmental philosophy
	Forecast changes in demand for the type and quantity of services
	Set objectives
	Develop strategies
	Design changes in the physical plant
	Plan new services, including satellite labs, Stat labs, or phlebotomy stations
	Prepare the budget
	Determine Stat lists, panic values, and a list of tests available on second and third shifts
Organizing and coordinating	Prepare a departmental table of organization
	Prepare position descriptions for each employee slot
	Assist in recruiting and selecting personnel
	Organize the work force and assign tasks
	Prepare work schedules
	Strengthen relationships with other hospital departments

Supervising   Indoctrinate new employees

Coach and counsel

Teach new methods and use of new instruments

Maintain discipline, safety, and morale

Achieve maximum productivity and quality

Controlling   Establish a reporting system by referring to the table of organization

Prepare standards of performance

Formulate and publish regulations, practices, policies, and procedures

Provide feedback to employees by coaching, counseling, and periodic formal performance reviews

Commend, reward, and promote

Maintain safety and discipline

Communicating Keep subordinates and superiors informed

Encourage input from employees

Keep open lines of communication with other departments

Motivating   Establish an atmosphere that satisfies employees' physical needs, increases productivity, and encourages self-development

Provide job enrichment

Encourage a positive work ethic

Developing subordinates	Evaluate employee skills, and assess educational, training, and experimental needs
	Provide necessary support to close employees' development gaps
	Delegate responsibility
	Encourage creativity
	Identify potential leaders, and plan succession
	Encourage continued formal education and participation in workshops and professional meetings
Self-development	Plan professional or managerial self-growth
	Keep up-to-date on professional, technical, and managerial matters
	Do personal research and development

Table 3-2. Dos and Don'ts in developing and using standards

Do	Don't
Make the list of duties complete, but not too long	Have too many or too few SPs for each duty
Group duties into major categories	Include responsibilities that aren't under the employee's control
Link SPs to duties and responsibilities	Put too much emphasis on behavior and attitude
Make the standards realistic, understandable, measurable, specific, and objective	Mix up levels of performance —some superior, some minimum
Be sure that both the employee and the supervisor know which level of performance the standards represent	Write unnecessary standards —repeating policy manuals, for example
Emphasize results	Base standards on invalid or unreliable data
Get input from the employee and others	Forget to update duties and SPs
Include negative standards to cover necessary constraints	
Inform employee of SPs and their significance	
Know who will match the performance with the standard	

40

References

1. Allan, P., and Rosenberg, S. Formulating usable objectives for manager performance appraisal. *Personnel Journal,* Nov. 1978, p. 626.

2. *A Workload Recording Method for Clinical Laboratories,* College of American Pathologists, Skokie, Ill. (published annually).

3. National Committee for Clinical Laboratory Standards, Villanova, Pa.

4. Alexander, J.O. Making managers accountable: Develop objective performance standards, *Management Review,* Dec. 1980, p. 43.

Suggested reading

Lawton, H.L., and Brownfield, R.L.: The number of personnel needed to perform examinations. *Health Laboratory Science,* April 1976, p. 118.

Sinton, E.B. What workload recording can do for you, *MLO,* Aug. 1978, p. 49.

Mack, D.J. Using workload statistics for manpower forecasting, *MLO,* Aug. 1978, p. 65.

Van Bokkelen, W.R. A case study on productivity improvement in a clinical laboratory setting. *In Examination of Case Studies on Productivity Improvements in the Clinical Laboratory,* American Hospital Association, Chicago, 1976, pp. 23-71.

Model Criteria For Peer Review, Competence Assurance Council, American Society for Medical Technology, Houston, 1981.

4

Implementation and follow-up

The format of performance standards is a matter of individual preference, but each standard should appear near the duty it refers to. This precludes a list of all duties followed by a still longer list of standards. One possibility is a two-column format with the duties on the left and standards on the right (Figure 4-1). An expanded version includes a third column for the names of observers (Figure 4-2). The form we use combines the duties and standards into sequential units. We designate duties by means of capital letters and standards by means of lower-case letters (Figure 4-3).

One essential task before you can implement performance standards is to get a solid commitment from your staff. Ask yourself.

● Do they understand the standards?

● Do they agree with them?

● Do they know what will happen if they fail to meet a standard?

If employees accept the idea without any arm-twisting, you can assume that they find it reasonable. If they help establish their own standards, all the better. You can be sure of their cooperation. In other words, the degree of compliance varies directly with the amount of employee input.

Ironing out an agreement on standards is like negotiating a work contract. The resulting document assures the supervisor that the work will be done as well as possible. The employee knows what is expected and is reassured that there won't be daily fluctuations in the demands placed on him.

Since for many of you this is the first attempt at designing a standards program, some SPs must remain tentative until you gain experience with the system. If failure to meet a standard will affect an employee's status, he should know what will happen. Will he return to an old assignment, lose a promotion, or be demoted or reassigned? The greater the risk, the more employees will push for lower standards.

On the other hand, you may have to loosen up with a nonassertive person or a new employe who doesn't want to get off to a bad start by displeasing you. You should also watch out for and temper the overenthusiastic type who sets unrealistically high goals.

Finally, review the position descriptions and performance standards with your superior. He or she may know of impending organizational changes that bear on the duties and standards, or find such barriers as budget restrictions or potential violations of labor laws or union contracts.

Follow-up

The first part of the postimplementation plan is to ensure that a standard is met. It's called checking — comparing actual performance with the standards. Checking answers these questions: Are employees doing what they are expected to do? Are they completing their tasks accurately and on time? Checking is actually the first step of the performance review, since it provides much information for that meeting. It also reveals the need for additional training.

The next part of follow-up is to maintain the credibility of your monitoring system through appropriate reviews. Keep a copy of each employee's standards, and review them occasionally. Tasks under your daily scrutiny are simple to monitor, but you may need to pay special attention to some of the others. Note reminders on your calendar, or keep a checklist close by.

45

One easy system is to use a standard desk calendar. After a performance review, enter the employee's name on the date when objectives are due. On each date, review the employee's personnel folder to find the objective and its SPs, then contact the employee if he has not achieved the objective. This often brings to light unanticipated constraints or barriers — or plain forgetfulness. Postponements may be necessary.

This approach not only is effective, but has the added advantage of letting subordinates know that you are aware of what is going on, and that you consider standards and objectives important — not an empty exercise. Provide positive and negative reinforcement for changes through daily coaching and, when necessary, counseling.

Encourage employees to report failures and obstacles. Congratulate them on completion of each objective or leg of an objective. This is a powerful motivational tool. Don't wait for the next formal performance review.

Be sure to let people know that duties and standards are not inscribed in stone. Modification, additions, and deletions are expected and encouraged. In fact, if the document is not used or not molded to individual needs, it will lose much of its benefit. It is often best to be tentative, especially if this is a new batch of standards. Set provisional criteria, and revise them as you gain experience. When standards or objectives prove to be unrealistic or inappropriate, they must obviously be modified; but give the employee time to adjust to the modification unless delays cannot be tolerated.

Additional applications of SPs

Once you have taken the first giant step, that of melding standards with duties and responsibilities, you're ready to take full advantage of this managerial tool. So far, we have emphasized the major function, providing the basis for constant performance feedback to employees. We've also mentioned the role of SPs in coaching, counseling, performance appraisals, and awarding promotions, merit-pay raises, and bonuses. You can also use SPs when you select employees for delegation, increased authority, and other forms of job expansion. Here are a few more ways to make the most of performance standards.

To indoctrinate new employees

Introduce new employees to the general use of SPs as part of their orientation. Build standards into your training strategy. Trainees appreciate knowing how well their new duties must be carried out, and they soon learn when to anticipate praise and when to expect criticism. They become aware of their shortcomings more readily and are more receptive to coaching and counseling. Positive attitudes gel during this formative phase.

To introduce new methods and instruments

With today's instrumentation and methodology in a constant state of flux, training is a routine part of laboratory life. This is an ideal time to familiarize everyone with the standards that must be met.

To emphasize the importance of a responsibility

Implicit expectations should be made explicit, and significant verbal expectations should be documented. This certainly applies to SPs. Here's an example: It had been an unwritten practice for our blood bank supervisor to provide the pathologist on weekend call with a list of administrative or professional problems — shortage of platelets, recipients with compatibility problems, and the like. The supervisor, who frequently was busy with other Friday afternoon chores, sometimes forgot to

47

write the memo. After this task was added to her position description with appropriate SPs, she rarely forgot it. What she had previously regarded as "nice but not important" assumed new meaning.

To increase performance by increasing challenge

SPs must be the same for all employees performing the same tasks. But what about providing challenge? One employee may struggle to attain a standard that another meets with ease. Avoid the temptation of raising that standard for the superior employee. Instead, encourage him or her to exceed the standard by a greater margin, and offer congratulations for doing so.

Questions and problems

Now we'd like to answer some questions that we've frequently been asked about our system of performance standards.

Where in the organization should SPs be introduced?

They should be used as far up the ladder as possible. Ideally, they would start with the chairman of the board and the chief executive officer. Realistically, they are more likely to be mandated at lower managerial levels, often without even providing appropriate guidelines or examples. The supervisors are usually not very happy about this, regarding it as another unnecessary administrative chore.

A good rule is that whoever decrees formulating SPs should prepare his own standards first. Employees should receive copies of this document after having been convinced that their jobs will be made easier by having performance criteria.

Hands-on workshops can be helpful in getting employees to appreciate the system and learn how to formulate their own standards.

How long does it take to develop SPs?

It should take no more than one to two hours to prepare the first draft for an employee, providing you have complete and up-to-date position descriptions. The first set is the most difficult and time-consuming. Since many employees in a laboratory section have fairly similar duties, their SPs will not differ greatly. So after the first one, the others are much easier to do. Where there are many diverse positions and the position descriptions are complex, more time is needed.

We completed SPs for all of our personnel over a 12-month period, using the date of each employee's performance review as the target date. None of the supervisors reported any difficulty in meeting this objective.

What do you do when an employee is not performing satisfactorily but is meeting all standards?

This one's obvious. Either your evaluation is wrong, or your SPs are incomplete or too low. We saw the same thing until our supervisors got used to the system. A supervisor might complain to her boss about an employee's performance. Told to look at the person's SPs, the supervisor might discover one of three possibilities: 1) the SPs do, in fact, state that performance at the employee's level is unacceptable; 2) the SPs give no standard for the task; or 3) the SPs provide a minimum standard, but the standard is too low.

If the first is true, the supervisor should have no trouble discussing the problem. If the second or third is the case, he must hold a counseling session and tell the employee that a new or higher standard is being introduced. This is essential—never slip in an SP without first discussing it with the employee.

Don't supervisors have to spend too much time monitoring the system?

Absolutely not. They actually spend less since employees do much of their own checking. At least we've found this to be true of most laboratory employees, especially the technologists. It isn't necessary to keep records of percentages and other figures or to have employees punch a time clock. Only when someone behaves unacceptably or is not performing up to expectations is it necessary to tally errors or omissions. If tardiness seems to be a problem, for example, then a record should be kept as to how often it occurs and how late the employee is. More serious deficiencies should always be documented.

A poor attitude is such a common problem and so subjective that special precautions are needed. Record what the employee did or didn't do that reflected the poor attitude. Write down actual quotes. Then when the inevitable confrontation takes place, you aren't at a loss to justify your accusation.

How rigidly do your supervisors enforce SPs?

Supervisors vary in applying SPs much as they do in other controlling functions. It depends largely on their leadership style. The hard-nosed autocrat has a tendency to follow SPs to the letter. Before SPs, employees complain that such bosses are overly critical and constantly looking over their shoulders. Afterward, such complaints should lessen because employees have in writing just what is and is not expected. They can tell when criticism is justified or petty. The autocratic leader's boss is also in a better position to challenge written expectations.

Lackadaisical supervisors, on the other hand, may ignore their employees' SPs. A laissez-faire style of leadership predisposes to this weakness. If if is permitted to continue, the SPs soon become worthless.

The rest of this book is devoted to practical examples of position descriptions, complete with duties, qualifications, levels of authority, and standards of performance. The examples range from laboratory director to technician, and they also cover such special positions as safety coordinator. They can, of course, be modified to suit your laboratory, and no doubt, there's plenty of room for improvement, too. We hope they will at least provide a solid base for your own, tailor-made documents.

Figure 4-1. A two-column display for duties and standards

Duty	Standards
To collect blood from inpatients	a. Morning rounds must be completed by 8 a.m.
	b. Stats and timed specimens must be collected within 10 minutes of the request.
	c. There must be no more than two multiple sticks or two unsuccessful venipunctures per day.
	d. There must be no more than one complaint per month from nurses, physicians, patients, or the laboratory staff.

Figure 4-2. A three-column format for duties and standards

Duty	Standards	Who checks/ When
To collect blood from inpatients	a. Morning rounds must be completed by 8 a.m.	Supervisor/daily
	b. Stats and timed specimens must be collected within 10 minutes of the request	Supervisor/daily
	c. There must be no more than two multiple sticks or two unsuccessful venipunctures per day.	Supervisor/daily
	d. There must be no more than one complaint per month from nurses, physicians, patients, or the laboratory staff.	Supervisor/daily

Figure 4-3. Duties and standards in sequential units

A. COLLECT BLOOD FROM INPATIENTS.

a) Morning rounds must be completed by 8 a.m.

b) Stats and timed specimens must be collected within 10 minutes of the request.

c) There must be no more than two mulitple sticks or two unsuccessful venipunctures per day.

d) There must be no more than one complaint per month from nurses, physicians, patients, or the laboratory staff.

Appendix A
Position descriptions and standards of performance

Key to examples of position descriptions and performance standards

Functions: Describes major categories of responsibilities.

Qualifications: Defines minimal qualifications of experience and education.

Reports to: Identifies the employee's immediate supervisor.

Supervises: Identifies personnel who report to the employee.

Coordinates with: Identifies members of other sections, departments, staff, or administrative personnel with whom the employee frequently works and communicates.

Authority: Describes what the employee is permitted to do. The class refers to the degree of authority.

Class 1: Full authority to take necessary action without consulting supervisor.

Class 2: Full authority as in Class 1, but the supervisor must be informed of the action taken.

Class 3: May present recommendations to the supervisor but must not take action until a decision is reached.

Column 1: Numerical sequence of all the employee's duties and responsibilities.

Column 2: The approximate percentage of time devoted to each duty.

Duties: Each duty is written in capital letters.

Performance standards: These follow each duty and are written in lower-case letters.

Note:
Unless otherwise noted, the following percentages serve as criteria:

Less than 75 percent of time = unsatisfactory performance.
More than 90 percent of the time = superior performance.

Position description — Clinical laboratory

Title: Laboratory director   **Section:** General laboratory
Shift: First   **Prepared by:** W. O. Umiker

Functions:

Provide a clinical diagnostic laboratory service.

Provide an anatomic pathology service.

Direct a blood bank and transfusion service.

Provide a cytology diagnostic service.

Qualifications:

Board-certified M.D. or D.O., CAP

At least three years' service as pathologist.

Previous administrative responsibilities.

Reports to:

Hospital medical director.

Supervises:

All clinical laboratory personnel. Directly supervises associate
pathologists, administrative assistant, education coordinator,
and supervisors of blood bank, chemistry and second and third
shifts.

Coordinates with:

Hospital administration, hospital department heads, medical
staff.

A. Patient care services (30%)

1 | 1%   **PROVIDE A CLINICAL DIAGNOSTIC LABORATORY SERVICE**

a) Services must include microbiology, hematology, chemistry, and immunohematology.

b) Turnaround times, quality, and range of services must be acceptable to medical staff.

c) Order-entry and results-reporting systems must be acceptable to the medical staff, nursing staff, and administration.

d) Manuals (or their equivalent) for requesting laboratory services, specimen collection, patient preparation, reference values, and other pertinent information for utilizing laboratory services shall be available, up-to-date, and acceptable to users.

e) Methodology, supplies, equipment, and procedure manuals must meet the approval of accrediting agencies.

f) Quality control must be acceptable to accrediting agencies and the medical staff.

Superior performance:

Written commendations.

Absence of valid written complaints from laboratory users, executive committee, medical staff, or administration.

Quality assurance results superior to those required for accreditation.

2 | 20%   **PROVIDE A SURGICAL PATHOLOGY SERVICE**

a) A pathologist will be available for O.R. diagnosis (frozen section) from 8 a.m. to 4:30 p.m., Monday through Friday, from 8 a.m. till noon on Saturday, and at other times by appointment.

b) Frozen section reports shall be ready within 15 minutes of receipt of the specimen, given by the pathologist directly to the surgeon, and recorded on the patient's chart while the patient is still in the O.R.

c) Less than 1 percent discrepancy (benign vs malignant) between frozen section reports and final pathological reports is acceptable.

d) Routine surgical pathology reports shall be completed within 24 hours of receipt of the specimen. When special procedures or consultations are needed, a preliminary written or verbal report must be given to the attending surgeon.

e) All surgical diagnoses will be coded by SNOMED (College of American Pathologists).

f) Slides, reports, and other appropriate materials shall be sent to pathology specialists when so requested by the attending surgeon or the patient.

g) No more than **three valid complaints** per year concerning accuracy of surgical pathology diagnosis is acceptable.

Superior performance:

No valid complaints from the president of the medical staff or the administration.

3 | 5% PROVIDE A CYTOLOGY DIAGNOSTIC SERVICE

a) Qualified cytotechnologist shall be available Monday through Friday.

b) Service includes gynecological, oral (Barr bodies),

57

urinary, respiratory tract, gastroesophageal, serous cavity fluid, cerebrospinal fluid, and thin-needle specimens.

c) Reports will be ready 24 hours following receipt of specimens (Monday through Thursday).

d) The percentage of false positives, false negatives, and "suspicious" reports shall be comparable to those reported by other medical centers.

e) No more than one valid complaint from users of the cytologic service per year is acceptable.

Superior performance:

No valid complaints from subscribers to the service.

4 4% **DIRECT A BLOOD BANK AND TRANSFUSION SERVICE**

a) Shall ensure an adequate supply of blood and blood products by establishing and maintaining a donor recruitment program or negotiating to contract with an outside agency.

b) Shall ensure an adequate inventory of blood and blood components, not only for the usual medical and surgical purposes, but also to meet the demands of a trauma service. The medical and surgical staff, transfusion committee, trauma committee and director of trauma service will determine the adequacy of the inventory.

c) The blood bank and transfusion service shall meet standards of AABB, JCAH, FDA, CAP, and any other accrediting agencies.

d) The blood bank shall be staffed by qualified personnel at all times.

e) Donor hours must be convenient for potential donors.

f) Turnaround time for preparing blood and blood products, both routine and emergency, must be satisfactory to physicians.

g) No more than one day's surgical schedule per year shall be canceled because of lack of blood or blood products.

h) There shall be no more than three valid complaints per year concerning turnaround time or the quantity of blood or blood components available.

i) There shall be no hemolytic transfusion reactions resulting from laboratory error.

j) Monthly transfusion service reports shall be made in writing to the transfusion committee.

k) A pathologist or other qualified physician shall be available for consultation regarding use of blood, selection of blood and blood products, and the investigation of transfusion reactions.

Superior performance:

Written commendations.

No canceled surgery or morbidity because of lack of blood or blood components.

No valid written complaints from donors, physicians, or others utilizing service.

Annual total number of donors greater than previous year.

More units of blood shipped out than received from other facilities.

Not on probation or services limited by any accrediting agency.

B. Human resource management and development (17%)

5	10%	**SELECT, DIRECT, AND CONTROL SUBORDINATES**

a) Sufficient personnel must be available at all times to handle the laboratory workload.

b) Work shall be supervised by qualified section and shift personnel supervisors.

c) The laboratory must meet or exceed all requirements of accrediting agencies.

d) Personnel turnover and attendance records must be equal to or better than those of other hospital departments.

e) Annual total salaries shall not exceed budget.

f) Safety requirements shall be met.

g) Licensure requirements shall be met.

Superior performance:

Commendations to hospital administration on the performance of lab personnel.

Personnel turnover and attendance records ranking among the top three hospital departments.

Personnel costs kept 5 percent or more below the amount budgeted.

6	1%	**PROVIDE AN ORIENTATION AND TRAINING PROGRAM FOR NEW EMPLOYEES**

a) The laboratory policy manual shall include a protocol that lists the steps for orienting and training new employees and a list of tasks for them to learn.

b) All new employees shall receive adequate orientation and training, with the lab director personally

supervising indoctrination of employees who report to him.

c) Completed report of orientation and training must
be signed by the trainer(s) and the trainee.

d) Personnel folders must include updated list of tests
or duties employees are qualified to perform.

e) No more than 10 percent of employee records shall
be deficient in any of the above.

Superior performance:

Over 95 percent of above records complete and up-
to-date.

Written favorable comments or commendations from
trainees or training supervisors.

No employee record deficient in indoctrination
program.

No valid written complaint from employee or supervisor relating to employee's not being capable of
performing test for which he is responsible.

| 7 | 6% | **PROVIDE A CONTINUING EDUCATION PROGRAM** |

a) The CE program shall meet standards of accrediting agencies and the hospital.

b) Sufficient funds will be budgeted for continuing
education and training of laboratory personnel,
subject to hospital-imposed financial restrictions.

c) There shall be no valid complaints, as determined
by the personnel director, from employees concerning lack of opportunities for CE or training.

d) Weekly meetings of the laboratory department,
laboratory sections, shifts, or office staff shall be

held for announcements and education. A record of such meetings will be included in monthly and annual laboratory reports.

e) Training in management will be available to supervisors or prospective supervisors.

f) A reference library must be maintained within the lab, meeting standards of the hospital medical library. Appropriate technical books and manuals must be available at the work benches.

g) A minimum continuing education requirement must be established for each category of employee. Over 80 percent of all employees shall meet this requirement.

Superior performance:

Over 90 percent of employees meet annual CE requirements.

No written valid complaints from employees concerning lack of opportunity to meet CE requirements.

C. Administration (19%)

8 6% PLANNING AND ORGANIZING

a) Goals and objectives shall be compatible with those of the hospital, as judged by the laboratory director's superior.

b) Policies, rules, and regulations must be appropriate, understandable, and complete, as judged by the laboratory director's superior. They must conform to those of the parent organization and not violate those of any government, accrediting, or regulatory agency.

c) Physical plant and staff sections must be organized to provide maximum efficiency.

d) Services will be scheduled with full consideration of need, cost, and regulatory priorities to the satisfaction of clinicians and administrators.

e) Accreditation standards and government regulations that apply to laboratory practice shall be fulfilled.

f) One- and five-year projections shall be made, covering organizational capability, changes in demand, and competitors' capabilities.

g) Shall determine feasibility and maintain fiscal responsibility in introducing changes.

h) Plans shall be submitted on schedule and in an acceptable format, and shall include specifics of a timetable, assignment of responsibilities, costs, and implementation.

i) Shall participate willingly in medical center plans to expand laboratory services in the hospital and in the community.

j) Time allocation to patient service, research, and education must be acceptable to administration.

Superior performance:

Administrative performance deemed superior by executive committee of the medical staff, administration, and director's chief.

9 2% FISCAL DUTIES

a) Productivity shall be equal or superior to other laboratories of similar type, based on CAP workload data.

b) Requests for space, equipment, services, and personnel must be reasonable and justified by documented data. Purchases based on cost-effectiveness, quality, and service. No more than one valid written complaint from purchasing department is acceptable.

c) Recommendations for salaries of laboratory personnel must be supported by salary ranges for similar jobs in competing laboratories or culled from regional reports.

d) Budget must be adhered to unless deviations are adequately justified.

e) Budget must be submitted on time.

f) Shall calculate and report costs of laboratory tests and recommended charges for services verifiable by finance department.

g) Shall compare relative costs of outside testing vs. in-hospital analysis and purchasing vs. leasing equipment.

h) Time-keeping records shall be submitted on time and contain no more errors than those of other departments. No more than three written valid complaints per year from the finance department.

i) Inventory control must be well organized with a continuing record of materials on hand, proper storage, and maintenance of levels that minimize waste, emergency requests, or shortfalls. There shall be no serious curtailment of service because of poor inventory control, and less than $1,000 per year loss from overstocking or poor environmental control.

Superior performance:

No written valid complaints from administration or finance department.

Commendations from superiors.

10	**5%**	**SELECT METHODS, SUPPLIES, AND EQUIP-MENT; ENSURE PROPER USE OF EQUIPMENT.**

a) No more than 10 percent of quality assurance deficiencies shall be attributable to obsolete or inadequate equipment, supplies, or methods.

b) No more than one interruption of service per month because of lack of back-up equipment or service is acceptable.

c) No more than three special requests for supplies per month is acceptable.

d) All downtime on major instruments must be recorded in the log.

e) Records shall indicate the quantity of supplies on hand.

f) Annual cost of supplies and equipment shall not exceed the budget.

Superior performance:

No QC deficiency because of equipment.

No interruptions of service.

No emergency requests for supplies.

Total cost of supplies and equipment at least 5 percent less than budgeted amount.

11	**1%**	**MAINTAIN LABORATORY SAFETY**

a) All hospital, local, state, and federal (OSHA) safety regulations shall be complied with.

b) Minor safety deficiencies will be corrected within 30 days; major ones immediately.

c) There will be no more than an average of one minor laboratory accident per month.

d) There will be no more than one accident per year that results in lost time.

e) Laboratory safety manual must be available and updated at least annually.

f) A qualified employee will be designated as laboratory safety coordinator. That employee will be a member of the hospital safety committee, and will have sufficient time to carry out safety inspections and prepare monthly reports.

Superior performance:

Safety deficiencies corrected within 10 days.

No lost time accidents per year.

12   3%   ESTABLISH AND MAINTAIN A QUALITY ASSURANCE PROGRAM

a) Q.A. program shall meet or exceed requirements of accrediting agencies including CAP, AABB, JCAH, FDA, and state Department of Health.

b) Deficiencies reported by on-site visits shall be corrected before deadline.

c) Laboratory and blood bank shall maintain all accreditations.

d) Cost of Q.A. program shall not exceed 25 percent of laboratory costs.

Superior performance:

Not placed on probation by any accrediting agency.

Cost of Q.A. program less than 20 percent of total laboratory expenses.

13   2%   RECORDS

a) Shall conform to hospital standards for data and systems control, forms control, computer applications, and results delivery.

b) Records shall be maintained in accordance with

hospital, government, and accrediting agency requirements.

D. Medical education (16%)

14 | 5% **INFORM MEDICAL STAFF OF NEW LABORATORY TESTS AND APPLICATIONS; PROVIDE CONSULTATIONS**

a) Shall prepare at least six laboratory bulletins per year dealing with new methods or interpretations.

b) Shall honor telephone and in-person requests by staff physicians for help in selecting or interpreting tests.

c) The laboratory service manual shall be updated at least annually; copies shall be distributed to all nursing floors and other service areas.

Superior performance:

Over 10 laboratory bulletins per year.

No valid complaints from medical staff.

15 | 6% **PROVIDE AN AUTOPSY SERVICE**

a) Autopsies shall be performed within 24 hours of receipt of authorized requests.

b) Record of pathological findings for death certificates must be provided at the completion of the autopsy. A list of gross anatomical findings shall be prepared within 24 hours of completion of the autopsy.

c) Final written reports shall meet JCAH, CAP, and other agency requirements. Final autopsy reports must include a narrative summary, gross and microscopic findings, and (except for medicolegal cases) a clinical-pathological correlation.

d) Final autopsy reports shall be completed within one week, unless special studies or consultations are required.

Superior performance:

No complaints from medical staff, medical records office, or funeral directors.

| 16 | 5% |

PARTICIPATE IN MEDICAL EDUCATION

a) Educational exercises such as CPC's or other medical presentations shall be provided when requested.

b) Participate in clinical department meetings when invited.

Superior performance:

No complaints from medical staff.

Written commendations.

E. Research and development (12%)

| 17 | 8% |

MAINTAIN PROFESSIONAL COMPETENCY

a) Be an active member of at least one national professional laboratory organization.

b) Meet the continuing education requirements of the AMA or CAP or equivalent.

c) Attend at least one workshop in pathology, blood banking, or management a year.

d) Maintain a written record of self-examination tests, such as ASCP Check Samples; document results in monthly QC laboratory reports.

Superior performance:

Maintain active membership in more than one national professional organization.

Exceed CE requirements of AMA or CAP by 50 hours a year.

Attend more than one professional workshop or meeting a year.

18 | 2% | DEVELOP APPROPRIATE METHODS AND INSTRUMENTATION

a) Methodology and instrumentation utilization shall be based on state-of-the-art feasibility and cost studies. Selection shall be confirmed by quality assurance studies that compare results with those of other similar laboratories.

19 | 2% | PARTICIPATE IN RESEARCH PROJECTS

a) Research activities must not interfere with responsibilities related to patient care, management, and teaching.

b) All research projects must be approved by the research committee.

c) Nonsubsidized projects utilizing laboratory space, equipment, and supplies must be approved by Administration.

Superior performance:

Obtain outside research grants.

Commendations and awards.

Publish professional papers.

Presentations to medical staff, professional organizations, and lay groups.

F. Medical staff duties (6%)

20 | 6% | SHALL BE MEMBER OF ACTIVE MEDICAL STAFF OF THE HOSPITAL

a) Shall perform all duties expected of a member of the medical staff to the satisfaction of the executive committee.

b) Shall serve as a member of the tissue, transfusion and trauma committees.

Superior performance:

Serve as an officer or committee chairman.

Be a member of more than three committees.

Exceed attendance requirement for committee meetings.

Position description—Clinical laboratory

Title: Chief medical technologist **Section:** General
Shift: First   **Pay grade:** 920 **Prepared by:** S. Yohe

Functions:

1. Supervise laboratory section supervisors.
2. Purchase and control of lab equipment and supplies.
3. Maintain laboratory quality control, safety, and data processing.
4. Financial management of lab.

Qualifications:

MT (ASCP) or equivalent (M.S. or M.A. preferred).

Six years' clinical laboratory experience; at least two in a supervisory position.

Reports to:

Laboratory director.

Supervises:

Section supervisors.

Coordinates with:

Lab office manager, nurse supervisors, hospital department heads, and physicians.

Limits of authority   **Class**

1. Institute quality control and safety measures.   2
2. Conduct on-site quality control and safety inspections in the laboratory.   1
3. Select new employees and authorize promotion for section supervisor positions.   3
4. Approve section supervisors' selection of new employees.   2
5. Recommend technologists for supervisory positions.   3
6. Assign duties and work hours to subordinates.   1
7. Schedule or approve vacations, holidays, and compensatory time off for oneself and subordinates.   1
8. Approve overtime.   2
9. Discipline subordinates.   3
10. Hear and act on minor grievances.   1
11. Select supplies for laboratory use.   1
12. Request outside maintenance services.   1
13. Select manufacturer and distributor of equipment.   3
14. Hold staff meetings.   1

A. Supervision (25%)

1 | 2% | PREPARE POSITION DESCRIPTIONS

a) Position descriptions and performance standards must be available on each employee and updated at least annually.

b) Position description and performance standards for new employees or new positions must be prepared before registering the vacancy.

c) Position description and performance standards must conform to laboratory norm in format and content.

2 | 5% | INTERVIEW, HIRE, AND PROVIDE INDOCTRINATION FOR NEW EMPLOYEES

a) Complete orientation of new employees must proceed according to prepared schedule and using standard format.

b) Completed documentation of orientation phase must be submitted at the completion of the orientation.

c) Orientation and training must be of a quality acceptable to the education coordinator and laboratory director.

3 | 5% | PROVIDE CONTINUING EDUCATION FOR EMPLOYEES

a) Must hold at least 10 meetings of subordinates per year.

b) Must submit documentation of these meetings to the education coordinator within two weeks following the meeting.

c) Employees must meet minimum CE credits required by the lab.

(1)	(2)	Duty/Performance Standards
4	**10%**	**COACH, COUNSEL, AND DISCIPLINE EMPLOYEES** a) Must hold and document counseling or disciplinary sessions as necessary. b) There must be no legitimate complaints regarding unfair or inappropriate treatment. c) Employees should express satisfaction during their performance reviews, with their supervisor's help.
5	**3%**	**HOLD PERFORMANCE REVIEWS** a) Must meet face-to-face with each subordinate at least annually to review performance based on standards established in the position description. b) The lab director must find the quality of evaluations satisfactory. c) Reports must be submitted to the lab office within one month of the employee's anniversary date. d) There must be no valid complaints from employees. e) Problems must be addressed as they occur, not saved for performance reviews.

B. Quality control (5%)

(1)	(2)	
6	**2%**	**REVIEW AND RECORD ALL QC AND MAINTENANCE** a) QC, maintenance, and downtime records must be available to the lab director upon his request 90 percent of the time.
7	**1%**	**PREPARE MONTHLY, QUARTERLY, AND ANNUAL QC REPORTS** a) Monthly reports must be submitted by the 20th of the following month 90 percent of the time. b) Quarterly reports must be submitted to the hospital quality assurance department by the due date.

c) Annual report must be submitted by July 31.

8 **<1%** **KEEP ABREAST OF NATIONAL, STATE AND OTHER REGULATIONS DEALING WITH QC**

a) Standards and regulations of the following agencies must be reviewed annually: department of health, CAP, and JCAH.

9 **<1%** **RECOMMEND MEASURES NECESSARY FOR LAB COMPLIANCE WITH ACCREDITING AGENCIES' STANDARDS**

a) Must notify section supervisors of changes in standards or requirements 90 percent of the time.

b) The lab director must be notified of a supervisor's failure to comply with QC recommendations.

10 **1%** **PREPARE AND PRESENT QC LECTURES**

a) Must present lectures in accordance with established education schedule.

b) Must present at least one general lab staff meeting on QC each year.

C. Safety (2%)

2% Note: If there's no safety coordinator, the chief medical technologist may have the safety responsibilities. See pages 113-117 for duties and standards.

D. Supplies and equipment (25%)

11 **10%** **OVERSEE INVENTORY CONTROL OF LAB SUPPLIES**

a) Must ensure an adequate amount of acceptable supplies for performance of all lab tests.

b) Must find adequate substitutes for supplies or reagents when necessary because of back orders, recalls, and the like.

(1)	(2)	Duty/Performance Standards
		c) There must be no excessive outdating because of overstocking, as judged by the lab director.
		d) There must be no more than four emergency requests per month because of understocking.
12	5%	**MEET WITH SALES AND TECHNICAL REPRESENTATIVES**
		a) Must contact or meet with company representatives to learn of new products and improvements in clinical lab products.
		b) Equipment must not be accepted for trial without proper authorization from the materials management department.
13	10%	**EVALUATE AND RECOMMEND LAB EQUIPMENT FOR PURCHASE OR LEASE**
		a) Equipment must not exceed approved capital budget; if it does, a documented budget exception form must be completed and approved.
		b) Equipment must be acceptable to the lab director and section supervisors.
		c) Cost analysis must be prepared and documented.

E. Research and development (20%)

(1)	(2)	
14	10%	**KEEP ABREAST OF NEW METHODS AND INSTRUMENTATION AS REQUESTED BY THE LABORATORY DIRECTOR**
		a) Must attend meetings or meet with technologists from other laboratories at least once a year to discuss new methods and instruments.
		b) Must undertake at least two new projects a year.
		c) At least 50 percent of the projects must culminate in a procedure or instrument being put into routine use in the lab.

d) New methods or instruments must prove to be wise selections in the lab director's judgment.

e) R&D projects must not interfere with administrative and technical responsibilities.

f) Projects must be completed by target date.

g) Budget must not be exceeded.

15 | 10%   DOCUMENT R&D PROJECTS AND OVERSEE TRAINING FOR ACCEPTED NEW METHODS AND EQUIPMENT

a) Statistical analyses and normal values must be determined before implementation.

b) Each employee's training record must be documented in personnel files.

c) The lab director must be notified of incomplete training.

F. Miscellaneous (23%)

16 | 5%   COMMUNICATE WITH NURSE SUPERVISOR TO DISCUSS LAB-NURSING PROBLEMS

a) Must meet at least quarterly.

b) A written report of the meeting must be submitted to the lab director within seven days.

c) Input from lab supervisors must be solicited before the meeting.

d) Problems encountered by the nursing staff must be discussed with the lab supervisor.

17 | <1%   OVERSEE ANNUAL BUDGET PREPARATION

a) Annual budget for laboratory must be submitted to the lab director one week before the deadline.

b) There must be no more than one valid complaint from supervisors concerning assistance rendered.

18 5% FACILITATE THE DEVELOPMENT, SELECTION, AND IMPLEMENTATION OF A DATA PROCESSING PROGRAM FOR THE CLINICAL LABORATORY

a) Must be done on a level satisfactory to the lab director and the hospital director of management information systems.

b) Must meet the established timetable set by personnel implementing the hospital computer system.

19 5% SELF-TRAINING AND DEVELOPMENT

a) Must attend at least two outside educational seminars per year.

b) Must attend a minimum of 75 percent of weekly laboratory meetings.

c) Must maintain an up-to-date CE record and attain at least the minimum required CE units.

20 8% OTHER DUTIES

NOTE: This position description is based on the assumption that the laboratory also has section supervisors. In a small lab, where the chief technologist is directly responsible for the bench techs, a position description can be formulated by combining the duties of the chief technologist with those of a bench supervisor.

Position description—Clinical laboratory

Title: Bench supervisor
Section: Hematology/Blood collection
Shift: First   **Pay grade:** 908   **Prepared by:** L. Dimter

Functions:

Supervise hematology, coagulation, and blood collection personnel.

Perform hematology and coagulation procedures.

Qualifications:

MT (ASCP) or equivalent.

Six years' clinical laboratory experience; at least two in hematology.

Reports to:

Associate pathologist.

Supervises:

Two full-time technologists, two part-time technologists, two full-time phlebotomists, seven part-time phlebotomists, students.

Coordinates with:

Other lab section supervisors, nurse supervisors, QC coordinator, safety coordinator, education coordinator, systems technologist, and office manager.

Limits of authority   **Class**

1. Select new employees in blood collection and
   hematology.   2

2. Assign duties and work hours to subordinates.   1

3. Schedule or approve vacations, holidays, and compen-
   satory time off for oneself and subordinates.   1

4. Call in extra help as needed, within budget limitations.   1

5. Approve overtime.   2

6. Sign out reports.   1

7. Discipline subordinates.   3

8. Hear and act on minor grievances.   1

9. Hold staff meetings.   1

10. Establish quality control criteria.   3

11. Reject unsatisfactory work of subordinates.   1

12. Request services of maintenance department.   1

13. Request outside maintenance services.   2

14. Select glassware, reagents, and other supplies.   1

15. Request services of safety, quality control, and education
    coordinators.   3

16. Establish or modify technical procedures.   2

17. Approve or establish safety measures in the section.   2

18. Select manufacturer and distributor of equipment.   3

19. Request typing assistance from office personnel.   1

20. Prepare budget for equipment and supplies.   2

A. Supervise hematology, coagulation, and phlebotomy services (70%)

1 2% PROVIDE COVERAGE FOR HEMATOLOGY SECTION

a) Shall ensure daily coverage from 7:30 a.m. to 4:30 p.m. at least 90 percent of the time.

b) Daily staffing shall be adequate to meet all standards and turnaround times.

2 2% PROVIDE COVERAGE FOR BLOOD COLLECTION

a) Shall ensure coverage of central collection area from 6:30 a.m. to 4 p.m., Monday through Friday, and 6:30 a.m. to 12 noon on Saturday at least 90 percent of the time.

b) Shall ensure coverage of the outpatient department's collection station 7 a.m. to 4:30 p.m., Monday through Friday, and 7 a.m. to 1 p.m. on Saturday at least 90 percent of the time.

c) Shall schedule collections outside of the hospital to the satisfaction of facilities served. No more than one valid complaint per year.

d) Shall ensure clean and pleasant collection areas.

e) Shall prepare and post weekend blood collection schedule.

3 2% REVIEW AND APPROVE ALL PROCEDURES IN SECTION

a) All new procedures shall be checked out before they are initiated.

b) All employees who will perform a procedure must be qualified to do so; this must be documented.

c) Before implementation, shall document with the QC coordinator that all new procedures have been investigated according to approved protocol.

d) Written procedure for each test (procedure sheet or card) must be readily available and legible and meet all requirements of accrediting agencies and our laboratory.

e) There shall be no more than two valid complaints per year about omitting any of the above.

| 4 | 2% | **PREPARE POSITION DESCRIPTIONS** |

a) Position descriptions and performance standards must be available on each employee and updated at least annually.

b) Position descriptions and performance standards for new employees or new positions must be prepared before registering the vacancy.

c) Position descriptions and standards of performance must conform to the laboratory norm as to format and content.

| 5 | 5% | **INTERVIEW, HIRE, AND INDOCTRINATE NEW EMPLOYEES** |

a) Shall complete orientation of new employees in both sections according to prepared schedule and using standard format.

b) Completed documentation of orientation phase must be submitted at the completion of the orientation program.

c) Shall make provisions for bench training in other sections and make sure it's completed on schedule.

d) Orientation and training phases must be of a quality acceptable to the education coordinator and pathologists.

| 6 | 3% | **PROVIDE BENCH-WORK INSTRUCTION** |

a) Shall schedule employees for reindoctrination

or retraining as requested by employees or supervisors.

b) Proficiency must be documented in employee records.

c) Shall initiate remedial benchwork instruction for employees who lack skills as indicated by observation or quality control results.

7	2%

ASSIGN AND MONITOR SPECIAL PROJECTS FOR EMPLOYEES

a) Shall periodically solicit employees' ideas for special work projects. If they are not forthcoming, shall recommend projects to employees.

b) Such projects shall be documented.

c) Shall provide valid reasons for noncompliance with above.

d) Every technologist must have a special assignment to be worked on when time permits.

8	5%

PROVIDE CONTINUING EDUCATION FOR EMPLOYEES

a) Shall hold at least ten section meetings per year.

b) Shall submit documentation of these meetings to the education coordinator within two weeks following meeting.

c) Employees must meet minimum CE credits required by the lab.

9	8%

SUPERVISE THE PERFORMANCE OF HEMATOLOGIC TESTS LISTED IN THE LAB SERVICE MANUAL

a) Daily PT, PTT, and CBCs without diffs must be reported by 9:30 a.m.

b) CBCs with diffs must be reported by 1:30 p.m.

c) All markedly abnormal results must be brought to the attention of the pathologist.

d) Results of abnormal differentials must agree with the pathologists' results to a degree acceptable to the reviewing pathologist.

e) Stat procedures must be reported within the established turnaround time.

f) Panic values must be called within 15 minutes of completion.

g) Routine testing must be completed by the end of the day or shift.

h) There shall be no more than four valid complaints a year from other shifts concerning work left for them.

10 1% MAINTAIN RECORD OF SECTION'S WORK HOURS

a) Accurate records must be submitted to the lab office by 8:30 a.m. on payroll Mondays.

11 2% COACH, COUNSEL, AND DISCIPLINE EMPLOYEES

a) Shall hold and document counseling or discipline sessions as necessary.

b) There shall be no legitimate complaints regarding unfair or inappropriate treatment.

c) Employees should express satisfaction with their supervisor's help in their performance reviews.

12 2% MAINTAIN SAFETY POLICIES AND PROCEDURES

a) There shall be no more than three safety deficiencies in the section per year.

b) Inspectors for accrediting agencies must report no more deficiencies than those in other lab sections.

c) There shall be no more than one accident per year.

13	**3%**	**HOLD PERFORMANCE REVIEWS**

a) Shall meet face-to-face with each employee in the section at least annually to review performance based on standards established in the position description.

b) Reviewing pathologist must find quality of evaluations satisfactory.

c) Reports must be submitted to the lab office one month before the employee's anniversary date.

d) There shall be no valid complaints from the employee.

e) Problems must be addressed as they occur, not saved for performance reviews.

14	**1%**	**PREPARE THE ANNUAL BUDGET**

a) The annual budget for equipment, supplies, and personnel shall be submitted to the lab director before the deadline.

b) Each new piece of equipment and any increase in the budget must be justified in writing.

c) Shall not exceed the budget in any category. Any variance must be explained in writing.

15	**2%**	**MAINTAIN LABORATORY SERVICE MANUAL**

a) Shall review at least annually the portion relating to hematology and ensure that appropriate changes have been made.

b) Shall document changes in procedures, normals, and the like as soon as they are introduced.

c) Information provided must meet the approval of the responsible pathologist and the lab director.

d) No more than three valid complaints a year from users of manual are acceptable.

85

16	**5%**	**MAINTAIN INVENTORY CONTROL**

a) An adequate amount of supplies must be on hand to perform tests.

b) Shall find an adequate substitute for supplies or reagents when necessary, as with backorders.

c) There must be no excessive outdating because of overstocking as judged by the pathologist responsible for the section.

d) There must be no more than one emergency request per month because of understocking.

17	**12%**	**MAINTAIN THE QUALITY OF WORK IN HEMATOLOGY**

a) Shall institute and maintain quality assurance measures as required by licensing and accrediting agencies or recommended by the QC coordinator or lab director.

b) Must achieve an annual QC record acceptable to licensing and accrediting agencies.

c) There must be no more deficiencies found during on-site inspections than in other lab sections.

d) A completed "Report of Deficiency Investigation" must be submitted to the lab director within 24 days of notification of deficiency.

18	**5%**	**MAINTAIN THE QUALITY OF WORK IN BLOOD COLLECTION**

a) The blood collection areas must be inspected at least weekly 90 percent of the time.

b) Problems must be investigated within 48 hours after a complaint has been registered.

c) There must be no more than six valid complaints per year from patients or physicians relating to blood collections.

d) There must be no more than three complaints per year from the lab director or supervising pathologist concerning the appearance or performance of the phlebotomists.

19   1%   MAINTAIN THE QUANTITY OF WORK

a) The CAP monthly report must be prepared and submitted to the administrative assistant by the seventh of each month.

b) The annual CAP productivity record must be equal to or higher than similar sections of hospitals of comparable size.

c) Valid complaints from medical and nursing staff must be no more frequent than those received by other sections, or more numerous than in previous years.

20   5%   MEET WITH SALES AND TECHNICAL REPRESENTATIVES

a) Visits of sales reps must be limited to less than 30 minutes unless special circumstances mandate more time.

b) Equipment must not be accepted for trial without proper authorization.

B. Perform hematologic and coagulation technical tasks (20%)

21   2%   ASSIST HEMATOLOGIST IN OBTAINING BONE MARROW SMEARS

a) Shall provide assistance at designated times.

b) Quality of smears must be acceptable to the hematologist.

22   18%   PERFORM PROCEDURES IN HEMATOLOGY AND COAGULATION

a) See 9 a-h.

87

C. Miscellaneous (10%)

23 | 10% | CONTINUING SELF-EDUCATION

a) Shall attend at least 50 percent of the weekly lab staff meetings.

b) Shall attend at least 75 percent of the weekly supervisors' meetings.

c) Shall maintain an up-to-date CE record and attain at least the minimum required CE units.

Position description—Clinical laboratory

Title: Technical supervisor   **Section:** Microbiology
Shift: First   **Pay grade:** 918   **Prepared by:** W. George

Functions:

Supervise the performance of employees in providing a diagnostic microbiology and serology service.

Perform routine and special microbiology and serology procedures.

Qualifications:

MT (ASCP), M.S. in clinical microbiology, or equivalent.

Reports to:

Associate pathologist.

Supervises:

Five full-time technologists, one part-time technologist, students.

Coordinates with:

Other laboratory supervisors, safety and QC coordinators, nurse epidemiologist, nurse supervisors, and office manager.

Limits of authority   **Class**

1. Establish and modify technical procedures.   2
2. Prepare budget for equipment and supplies.   2
3. Discipline personnel in the section.   3
4. Sign out reports.   1
5. Recommend employees for CE programs.   3
6. Evaluate microbiology bench supervisor, and review evaluations of other personnel in the section.   2
7. Select or reject new employees to be assigned to the section.   2
8. Accept and act on grievances.   2
9. Initiate special studies as needed.   2
10. Select equipment and supplies.   1
11. Approve duties and work hours of subordinates.   1
12. Call in extra help as needed, within budget limitations.   1
13. Approve overtime.   2
14. Hold staff meetings.   1
15. Establish quality control criteria.   3
16. Reject subordinates' unsatisfactory work.   1
17. Request services of the maintenance department.   1
18. Request outside maintenance services.   2
19. Request services of safety, quality control, and education coordinators.   3
20. Approve or establish safety measures.   2
21. Request typing assistance from office personnel.   1

A. Supervision (20%)

(1)	(2)	
1	<1%	**PLAN OWN POSITION DESCRIPTION, AND PREPARE FOR AN ANNUAL EVALUATION**

a) Shall review position description at least annually.

b) Standards must be acceptable to supervisor.

c) Shall submit an annual performance report 25 days before anniversary of employment date.

d) Performance evaluation shall be reviewed with the education coordinator, as it relates to teaching duties, before being submitted to supervisor.

2	3%	**REVIEW THE ANNUAL PERFORMANCE APPRAISAL AND POSITION DESCRIPTIONS OF EMPLOYEES IN THE SECTION**

a) Shall review each position description once a year when the performance appraisal is due.

b) Reviewing pathologist must find them satisfactory.

c) The position description and standards must conform to the laboratory norm as to format and content.

d) Reports must be submitted to the lab office one month before the anniversary date of the employee.

3	7%	**MAINTAIN PRODUCTIVITY AND QUALITY OF THE SECTION**

a) Annual productivity, as measured by the CAP, shall equal or exceed the productivity figures of other hospitals our size in both microbiology and immunology.

b) Proficiency test specimens, as submitted by ASCP, CAP, and state health department, shall show results equal to or better than the agencies' minimal acceptable performance.

c) Shall sign out all microbiology and immunology reports, checking for correctness, legibility, and neatness.

d) Shall ensure adequate staffing to meet all standards and turnaround times.

4 | 3% | COACH, COUNSEL, AND DISCIPLINE EMPLOYEES IN THE SECTION

a) Shall act promptly on complaints and problems.

b) There shall be no legitimate complaints regarding unfair or inappropriate treatment.

c) Employees should express satisfaction with their supervisor's help in performance reviews.

5 | 2% | PREPARE THE SECTION'S ANNUAL BUDGET

a) The budget for expenses, revenue, and equipment shall be submitted to the laboratory director before the deadline.

b) Expenditures shall be within budget except when special permission has been obtained from the laboratory director.

c) Each new piece of equipment and any increase in the budget must be justified in writing.

6 | 2% | MAINTAIN EFFECTIVE COMMUNICATION WITHIN AND OUTSIDE THE DEPARTMENT

a) The laboratory service manual coordinator shall be notified of problems or changes in procedures that affect other departments.

b) The pathologists and laboratory section supervisors shall be notified of problems or changes in procedures that affect their sections.

| 7 | 2% | **DELEGATE RESPONSIBILITIES AND DUTIES TO EMPLOYEES IN THE SECTION** |

a) Shall assign duties and responsibilities to bench supervisor and technologists when appropriate.

| 8 | 1% | **MAINTAIN LABORATORY SERVICE MANUAL** |

a) Shall review at least annually the portion relating to microbiology and ensure that appropriate changes have been made.

b) Shall document changes in procedures, normals, and the like as soon as they are introduced.

c) The information provided must meet the approval of the responsible pathologist and the lab director.

d) No more than three valid complaints a year from users of the manual are acceptable.

B. Technical and professional reports (9%)

| 9 | 2% | **PREPARE ANTIBIOGRAM** |

a) An antibiogram shall be calculated annually for organisms isolated in our hospital.

b) Results shall be printed and distributed to all staff physicians and nursing stations.

| 10 | 4% | **PREPARE SNOP REPORT** |

a) Shall calculate SNOP report from section records and submit it to the lab office no later than the 10th of each month.

b) Shall review results for trends or problems and act accordingly.

| 11 | 3% | **PREPARE SPECIAL REPORTS** |

a) A contaminated clean-catch urine report shall be prepared on one month's data by May of each year.

b) Blood cultures shall be monitored monthly, noting

1) the contamination rate; 2) the rate of multiple organism infections; 3) the rate of positives; and 4) the rate of anaerobic isolates.

c) Reports shall be prepared as needed or assigned by the pathologists.

C. Teaching (35%)

12 | 20% | **LECTURE TO STUDENTS IN MICROBIOLOGY AND SEROLOGY**

a) The lecture schedule shall be reviewed and, if necessary, revised annually.

b) Notes and objectives shall be reviewed at least 10 days before class with necessary revisions typed by the school secretary.

c) The education coordinator shall receive the exam questions at least one week before the exam date.

d) There shall be no more complaints about teaching than the average received by all other lab instructors.

13 | 10% | **TEACH BASIC BENCH WORK**

a) The basic bench-work schedule shall be reviewed and, if necessary, revised annually.

b) Shall arrange for necessary supplies for student basic lab.

c) Shall construct, administer, and grade examination at end of basic lab.

14 | 5% | **OVERSEE STUDENT MICROBIOLOGY AND SEROLOGY BENCH-WORK PROGRAM AND TEACHING, INCLUDING THE FINAL EXAMINATION AND EVALUATION**

a) Bench-work schedules shall be reviewed, and if necessary, revised annually.

b) A bench-work evaluation interview shall be conducted with each student upon completion of rotation.

c) The education coordinator must receive final grades and evaluation forms no later than 10 working days after the completion of the rotation.

D. Continuing education and training (10%)

15 | 4% | TRAINING AND DEVELOPMENT OF SECTION PERSONNEL

a) Shall hold and record at least 10 section meetings a year.

b) Shall submit documentation of these meetings to the education coordinator within two weeks following meeting.

c) Each employee in the section shall attend at least one outside professional meeting per year.

d) Each employee must achieve the minimum required CE units per year.

e) Each employee must attend at least half of lab staff meetings.

f) When requested, shall provide practical indoctrination for new employees' orientation.

16 | 4% | SELF-DEVELOPMENT AND TRAINING

a) Shall attend at least two outside meetings per year.

b) Shall attend at least 75 percent of laboratory meetings. These include supervisors', CE, instructors', and section meetings.

c) Shall maintain an up-to-date CE record and attain at least the minimum required units.

17 | 2% | INFECTION SURVEILLANCE

a) Shall serve on the hospital infection surveillance

committee and attend at least 75 percent of the meetings.

b) Shall alert the hospital epidemiologist or the committee of any potential nosocomial infection problems noted by the laboratory.

E. Research and development (20%)

18 | 17% **INTRODUCE OR REVIEW AND APPROVE ALL NEW PROCEDURES IN THE SECTION**

a) Shall introduce at least one new procedure a year.

b) Shall approve all new procedures before evaluation and initiation.

c) Shall follow the new procedure protocol.

d) The section procedure manual shall be reviewed at least annually.

e) Shall ensure that all employees who will perform the procedures are qualified to do so; this must be documented.

f) Written procedure for each test (procedure sheet or card) must be readily available and legible and meet all requirements of accrediting agencies and our laboratory.

g) There shall be no more than two valid complaints per year on omitting any of the above.

19 | 3% **MEET WITH SALES AND TECHNICAL REPRESENTATIVES**

a) Meet with company representatives to learn of new products and improvements in clinical microbiology and serology products.

b) Equipment shall not be accepted for trial without proper authorization.

F. Miscellaneous (5%)

20 — **SAFETY**

a) Shall ensure that the entire section follows all
hospital and laboratory policies and procedures.

b) There shall be no more than three safety deficiencies per year.

c) Inspectors for accrediting agencies shall report no
more deficiencies than those in other lab sections.

d) There shall be no more than one accident per year.

21 — **ATTENDANCE**

a) The section's absentee rate shall not exceed a rate
acceptable to the lab director.

22 5% **BENCH WORK**

a) Shall do routine bench work when workload or
shortage of personnel justify it.

Position description—Clinical laboratory

Title: Medical technologist   **Section:** Microbiology
Shift: First   **Pay grade:** 902   **Prepared by:** J. Reider

Functions:

Perform and interpret routine diagnostic microbiology procedures.

Perform and interpret routine diagnostic serology procedures.

Instruct MT students in routine bacteriology.

Qualifications:

M(ASCP), MT(ASCP), or equivalent.

Reports to:

Microbiology bench supervisor.

Supervises:

Students.

Coordinates with:

Other section personnel, education coordinator.

Limits of authority	**Class**
1. Perform repeat tests when results are questionable.	2
2. Judge adequacy of submitted specimens, and request additional specimen if necessary.	1
3. Modify work patterns to facilitate daily workload.	1
4. Organize bacteriology bench-work teaching.	2

A. Microbiology tests (50%)

1 | 35% **PERFORM ROUTINE BACTERIOLOGY PRO-
CEDURES INCLUDING READING OF PLATES,
IDENTIFICATION, AND ANTIBIOTIC SUSCEPTI-
BILITY TESTING OF SUSPECTED PATHOGENS**

a) Cultures must be planted on appropriate media
within 15 minutes of receiving the specimens.

b) Stat Gram stains must be prepared and interpreted
within 30 minutes of receiving the specimen.

c) Plates must be read and necessary tests set up by
3 p.m.

d) Must advise technicians on identification workup
of unusual isolates.

e) All procedures in the department must be performed according to laboratory specifications.

f) There shall be no more than three complaints (incident reports) a year from physicians or nursing
personnel regarding bacteriology results and
procedures.

2 | 4% **PERFORM ROUTINE AFB WORK INCLUDING
SPECIMEN PROCESSING AND STAINING**

a) Process, culture, and prepare smears of specimens
within one hour.

b) Interpret stains within 15 minutes, and notify the
proper authorities when positive.

3 | 2% **PERFORM ROUTINE MYCOLOGY INCLUDING
SPECIMEN PLANTING AND VARIOUS
STAINING PROCEDURES**

a) Smears of specimens must be cultured and prepared
within 15 minutes.

b) Gram stains, India ink, and KOH preparations must
be prepared and interpreted within 30 minutes.

4	5%	**PERFORM ROUTINE PARASITOLOGY WORK INCLUDING SPECIMEN PROCESSING, STAINING PROCEDURES, AND PARASITE IDENTIFICATION**

a) Specimens must be examined and placed in preservatives within 10 minutes.

b) Direct smears must be prepared and interpreted within 15 minutes.

c) Stained smears must be prepared and interpreted within two hours.

d) Concentration of specimens must be completed within one hour.

5	2%	**REPORT RESULTS**

a) Written reports must be legible, neat, and accurate 85 percent of the time.

b) Reports must include date, initials of the technologist, and the time the specimen was planted or processed.

c) Stat reports, positive blood and CSF culture, and other necessary results must be called and this action noted on the report form.

6	2%	**PERFORM MICROBIOLOGY QUALITY CONTROL**

a) There shall be no more than one complaint per year.

b) QC results must be recorded on appropriate sheets, dated, and initialed.

c) Supervisor must be notified of out-of-control results.

B. Serology tests (12%)

7	10%	**PERFORM ROUTINE AND SPECIAL SEROLOGY PROCEDURES**

a) These procedures must be performed within the

stated turnaround time at least 85 percent of the time.

b) Must learn new procedures as they are added.

c) There shall be no more than three complaints per year from physicians or nursing personnel regarding serology results and procedures.

| 8 | 1% | **REPORT RESULTS**

a) Written reports must be legible, neat, and accurate 85 percent of the time.

b) Reports must note whether the specimen is satisfactory or unsatisfactory, and be dated and initialed.

c) Stat or call-results reports and other necessary results must be called and noted on the report form.

| 9 | 1% | **PERFORM SEROLOGY QUALITY CONTROL**

a) There shall be no more than one complaint per year.

b) QC results must be recorded on the appropriate sheets, dated and initialed.

c) The supervisor must be notified of out-of-control results.

C. Skin tests (2%)

| 10 | 2% | **ADMINISTER INTRACUTANEOUS SKIN TESTS**

a) Must inject one skin test within 10 minutes.

b) The test must be given in accordance with standard operating procedure.

c) There shall be no more than one complaint per year from physicians or nursing personnel regarding the administration of skin tests.

D. Bench-work teaching (25%)

11 | 25% **TEACH ROUTINE BACTERIOLOGY
TO STUDENTS**

a) Students must be instructed according to prepared
   schedule.

b) The final grade must be calculated and given to the
   technical supervisor within one week after the
   student finishes rotation.

c) There must be no more than three complaints per
   year from students or the education coordinator
   regarding teaching.

E. Special assignments (5%)

12 | 3% **PERFORM SPECIAL PROJECTS
ASSIGNED BY SUPERVISOR**

a) The project must be completed within the agreed-
   upon time limit 75 percent of the time.

13 | 2% **DO CAP AND OTHER PROFICIENCY SURVEY
SPECIMENS AS ASSIGNED**

a) These specimens must be completed on schedule
   at least 95 percent of the time.

b) There shall be no more than three unacceptable
   results per year.

F. Miscellaneous (6%)

14 | 6% **ACHIEVE AT LEAST THE MINIMUM
CONTINUING EDUCATION CREDITS**

a) Must attend at least 50 percent of laboratory staff
   and section meetings.

b) Must attend required hospital meetings.

c) Must attend one outside meeting in the field of
   microbiology or serology per year.

15	—	**MAINTAIN ATTITUDE AND MORALE**

a) There must be no more than one valid complaint per year from other laboratory personnel regarding cooperation.

b) There must be no more than one safety violation per year.

c) Annual sick time must be equal to or better than the laboratory average.

d) Must return from lunch and breaks promptly.

e) Must report to work on schedule 95 percent of the time.

f) Must remain after hours at the request of the technical supervisor to complete work 80 percent of the time requested.

Position description—Clinical laboratory

Title: Medical technologist   **Section:** Chemistry
Shift: First   **Pay grade:** 902   **Prepared by:** R. Serfass

Functions:

Perform routine and special diagnostic chemical procedures and routine urinalysis.

Perform diagnostic procedures in other sections.

Serve as general lab supervisor on weekends and holidays.

Qualifications:

MT(ASCP), C(ASCP), or equivalent.

Reports to:

Chemistry bench supervisor.

Supervises:

Lab employees on weekends and holidays.

Students and trainees.

Coordinates with:

Other section personnel.

Limits of authority   Class

1. Order or perform repeat tests when results are questionable.   2

2. Judge adequacy of submitted specimen; request additional specimen if unsatisfactory.   1

3. Call in backup personnel on evening and weekend shifts when workload requires it.   2

4. Standard supervisory authority when serving as supervisor on weekends or holidays.   1

A. Chemistry tests (85%)

1 | 75% | PERFORM TESTS ON THE CHEMISTRY AND URINALYSIS PROCEDURE LIST

a) Must learn new procedures added to the test list.

b) Procedures must be performed within the stated turnaround time at least 90 percent of the time.

c) Must analyze QC data for each procedure, record values on appropriate log sheets, and report to the supervisor when results are outside two standard deviations.

d) There must be no more than three complaints (incident reports) per year from physicians or nursing personnel regarding personally performed procedures.

2 | 4% | TRANSCRIBE TEST RESULTS ON THE REPORT FORM

a) Report must include technologist's initials.

b) Results must be legible and neat.

c) Report must include information regarding abnormal appearance of specimen or be marked satisfactory.

d) Abnormal results must be circled.

3 | 1% | REPORT PANIC VALUES OR TO-BE-CALLED RESULTS BY TELEPHONE

a) Call panic value or to-be-called results within 15 minutes of test completion.

b) Report must document that result was called and when it was done.

4 | 5% | PERFORM DESIGNATED QC PROCEDURES

a) There must be no more than two valid complaints per year from supervisor.

(1)	(2)	
		b) Log books must be signed when performing QC procedures at least 90 percent of the time.
		c) Corrective action for QC problems on KDA must be reported at least 90 percent of the time.
5	—	**NOTIFY THE BENCH SUPERVISOR WHEN SUPPLIES, TEST KITS, OR REAGENTS SHOULD BE REORDERED**
		a) There must be no more than two lapses per year.

B. Tests in other lab sections (10%)

(1)	(2)	
6	5%	**PERFORM ROUTINE PROCEDURES IN OTHER SECTIONS, AS REQUIRED FOR WEEKENDS AND HOLIDAYS**
		a) Quality of work and productivity must meet minimal standards for personnel who ordinarily perform this work.
		b) There must be no more than two valid complaints per year from supervisory personnel.
7	5%	**COLLECT BLOOD SPECIMENS**
		a) There must be no more than one complaint per year from nurses, physicians, or phlebotomy supervisor concerning method of blood collection, attitude, or courtesy to patient.

C. Supervisor assignment (5%)

(1)	(2)	
8	5%	**SUPERVISE LABORATORY PERSONNEL ON WEEKENDS AND HOLIDAYS**
		a) Routine procedures (CBC, biochemical screen, PT and PTT, electrolytes) must be reported by the deadlines listed in the laboratory procedure manual.
		b) Stat procedures must be completed within established turnaround times.

c) Routine work must be completed before leaving.

d) Backup personnel must be called in when needed.

e) Overtime must be justified to the satisfaction of the lab director.

f) There must be no more than two valid complaints from medical staff, nursing service, supervised employees, or section supervisors concerning the laboratory work done on the shift supervised.

D. Miscellaneous

9 — **MAINTAIN ATTITUDE AND MORALE**

a) There must be no more than one valid complaint per year from other lab personnel regarding co-operation.

b) There must be no more than one safety violation per year.

c) Annual sick time must be equal to or better than laboratory average.

d) Must return from lunch and breaks promptly.

e) Must report to work on schedule 95 percent of the time.

f) Must remain after hours at the request of the technical supervisor to complete work 80 percent of the time requested.

Position description—Clinical laboratory

Title: Cytotechnologist   **Section:** Histopathology
Shift: 7:30 a.m.-4:30 p.m.   **Pay grade:** 090
Prepared by: Dr. Eisenhower

Functions:

Screen cytologic smears for malignant cells, hormone levels, and microorganisms.

Prepare and stain cytologic preparations.

Qualifications:

CT(ASCP) or equivalent with two years' experience in exfoliative cytology.

Reports to:

Histopathology supervisor.

Supervises:

No one.

Coordinates with:

Staff pathologists, QC and safety coordinators, laboratory office typists. Radiology personnel and physicians (thin-needle preparations).

Limits of authority   **Class**

	Limits of authority	Class
1.	Modify cytologic techniques.	3
2.	Reject cytology specimens that do not meet established standards.	1
3.	Request additional specimens when those submitted are inadequate.	1
4.	Give preliminary verbal reports to physicians.	1
5.	Sign out final interpretation of negative GYN cytology reports (except the 10% reviewed by pathologists).	1

A. Process cytological smears (15%)

1 | 15% | REGISTER, SELECT PARTICLES, CONCENTRATE, FILTER, SMEAR, MOUNT, STAIN, AND COVERSLIP

a) Specimens must be processed according to procedure manual.

b) Smears must be acceptable to pathologist.

c) There must be no more than three valid complaints from physicians per year in preparation of aspiration cytology preps.

d) There must be no more than three documented complaints per year concerning quality of smears.

e) There must be no more than three valid complaints per year concerning the appearance of the benchwork area.

B. Screen cytology smears (80%)

2 | 80% | IDENTIFY ABNORMAL CELLS, FUNGI, PARASITES, VIRAL CHANGES, BARR BODIES, AND HORMONAL CHANGES IN SMEARS

a) An average of 60 slides must be screened per day.

b) Negative GYN reports must be signed out before the end of the shift.

c) All non-GYN smears and 10 percent of negative GYN smears must be submitted for review by pathologists.

d) Must call no more than 5 percent of smears positive or suspicious when the pathologist interprets them as negative.

e) Must call no more than 3 percent of smears negative when the pathologist interprets them as positive or suspicious.

f) Must correctly identify fungi, parasites, or viral changes.

C. Miscellaneous (5%)

3 <1% OBTAIN BUCCAL SMEARS FROM PATIENTS

a) Buccal smears must contain sufficient cells for interpretation.

b) There must be no more than one valid complaint per year from a patient or physician.

4 <1% MAINTAIN QUALITY CONTROL

a) Must keep an up-to-date log of all abnormal cytology results.

b) Monthly productivity records must be submitted to the supervisor by the fifth of each month.

c) Quality of work must average at least "good" on an unsatisfactory-poor-good-excellent scale.

d) There must be no more than one unsatisfactory or two poor QC reports per month.

e) Must participate in cytology Check Sample and other outside QC exercises. Interpretations must be acceptable to the pathologist.

5 <1% MAINTAIN SAFETY

a) There must be no more than two reported incidents per year.

b) Must attend all safety programs required by the laboratory and hospital.

6 4% MAINTAIN CONTINUING EDUCATION

a) Must attend at least one outside professional seminar per year.

b) Weekly staff meeting minutes must be read and initialed.

c) Must study cytology Check Sample reports.

d) Must read one cytology journal regularly or selected cytology articles from other journals.

e) All cytology Check Samples must be completed within a week of receipt.

f) Must give one staff meeting and two student lectures per year.

g) Must attain minimum CE credits required by the lab.

7 — MAINTAIN ATTITUDE AND MORALE (SEE PAGES 98-103)

Position description—Clinical laboratory

Title: Safety coordinator (part-time)
Section: General laboratory
Shift: First   **Pay grade:** 905   **Prepared by:** P. Welk

Functions:

Keep laboratory under surveillance for safety violations.

Advise laboratory employees on safety regulations and practices.

Qualifications:

MT (ASCP) or equivalent with two years' experience in the clinical laboratory.

Minimum of 10 hours' instruction or training in laboratory safety.

Familiarity with safety regulations applicable to clinical laboratories.

Reports to:

Associate pathologist.

Supervises:

No one.

Coordinates with:

Laboratory director, laboratory section supervisors, hospital staff medical officers, and hospital safety committee.

Limits of authority   **Class**

1. Inspect laboratory areas at any time.   1

2. Question laboratory personnel, hospital employees in the lab, and visitors concerning activities relating to safety.   1

3. Report safety violations to hospital safety committee or higher management if remedial action is not instituted by lab management.   2

4. Recommend laboratory tests on personnel to determine effectiveness of preventive measures, or to investigate safety problems.   3

5. Send laboratory personnel to emergency room in accidents causing personal injury.   2

A. Provide safety surveillance (65%)

1 | 20% | CONDUCT SAFETY INSPECTIONS IN LABORATORY

a) At least 11 general lab inspections must be completed per year.

b) Inspection deficiencies must be submitted to the supervisor within two days of the inspection.

c) Deficiencies must be followed up within two weeks to see if they have been corrected.

d) An exception statement must be submitted to the supervisor when the two-week correction deadline can't be met.

e) Must investigate any suspected health hazard to lab personnel as soon as the report is received.

2 | 10% | PREPARE LABORATORY SAFETY REPORTS

a) A monthly safety report must be submitted by the 15th of the following month. The report must include inspection results, deficiency corrections, new policies and equipment, staff meeting announcements, continuing education, and safety incidents.

b) An annual report must be submitted within two weeks before the end of the fiscal year.

c) Safety deficiencies or violations, injuries, or employment-related illness must be reported when known.

3 | 35% | MAINTAIN LABORATORY SAFETY MANUALS

a) Written policies and procedures must be acceptable to the supervisor and in accordance with current CAP, OSHA, JCAH, and state regulations for laboratory safety manuals.

b) Laboratory section policy manuals must not violate safety rules.

115

c) Manuals must be reviewed annually.

B. Safety consultant and inspector (30%)

4	**20%**	**EDUCATE EMPLOYEES AND STUDENTS IN LABORATORY SAFETY**

a) New safety information must be posted.

b) A safety program must be presented at the laboratory staff meeting twice a year.

c) A safety announcement must be presented at the staff meeting at least twice per month.

d) Indoctrination of new employees or students in lab safety must be completed within two weeks of their starting date.

e) Must present a lab section meeting on safety when requested.

f) Must question employees randomly to determine their safety knowledge and safety education needs. Findings must be included in monthly report.

5	**5%**	**SERVE AS A SAFETY CONSULTANT TO LABORATORY MANAGERS**

a) Must demonstrate familiarity with current CAP, OSHA, JCAH, and state safety requirements.

b) There must be no more than one valid complaint per year from the supervisor, lab director, or hospital safety committee relating to the safety coordinator's ignorance of safety regulations.

c) There must be no more than one safety violation during an outside agency's inspection that is attributable to ignorance of laws and regulations.

d) There must be no more than one valid complaint per year from supervisors because of a failure to prepare employees' safety records for performance reviews.

6	4%	**ATTEND HOSPITAL SAFETY COMMITTEE MEETINGS**

a) Must represent the laboratory at meetings. If unable to attend, must notify the chairman at least one day before the meeting.

b) Must attend at least 75 percent of these meetings.

c) Must report pertinent meeting information to the appropriate superior.

d) There must be no more than one valid complaint per year from a superior or the chairman of the hospital safety committee.

7	1%	**ATTEND PROFESSIONAL SAFETY MEETINGS**

a) Must attend at least one outside safety meeting every two years.

C. Miscellaneous (5%)

8	5%	**PERFORM MISCELLANEOUS DUTIES**

a) Must perform and record face-velocity checks of safety hoods and fume hoods once a month.

b) Must perform and record an eyewash check once a month.

c) Must perform and record a monthly check on random electrical outlets and wires.

d) Must ensure that hepatitis and tuberculosis testing is done annually on all lab employees and must maintain a record of the results.

e) Must record annual chest x-rays of microbiology personnel.

Position description—Clinical laboratory

Title: Senior phlebotomist   **Section:** Blood collection
Shift: 6:30 a.m.-3 p.m.   **Pay grade:** 052
Prepared by: L.Dimter

Functions:

Perform phlebotomies on inpatients and outpatients.

Organize blood collection work.

Process blood specimens.

Police blood collection work area.

Train new employees and students.

Qualifications:

Two years' experience as a phlebotomist.

Licensed car driver.

Reports to:

Supervisor of hematology and blood collection.

Supervises:

Students and new employees during orientation.

Coordinates with:

Floor nurses, laboratory supervisors, and laboratory office personnel.

Limits of authority	Class
1. Organize workload in the blood collection area.	1
2. Schedule blood collection outside the hospital.	1
3. Supervise students and new employees during their blood collection orientation.	1

A. Blood collection (70%)

1 | 50% **COLLECT BLOOD FROM HOSPITAL INPATIENTS AND OUTPATIENTS**

a) Morning rounds must be completed by 8 a.m.

b) Stats and timed requests must be done within 10 minutes.

c) Repeat venipuncture rate must not be higher than 5 percent of total venipunctures.

d) Unsuccessful venipunctures must not be higher than 5 percent of total venipunctures.

2 | <1% **COLLECT BLOOD AT NURSING HOMES AND PRIVATE HOMES (AS NEEDED)**

a) Must maintain active driver's license.

b) There must be no more than three unsuccessful venipunctures per month.

c) There must be no more than three valid complaints per year from patients or nursing home personnel.

3 | 20% **ORGANIZE WORKLOAD OF BLOOD COLLECTION AREA**

a) Must correctly prepare slips for early morning rounds.

b) Must assign phlebotomists' itineraries with no more than one complaint per month for failure to respond within turnaround times.

B. Specimen processing (15%)

4 | 5% **DELIVER SPECIMENS TO LABORATORY SECTIONS**

a) Specimens must be delivered within 30 minutes of their arrival in the lab.

119

b) Stat specimens must be delivered within five minutes.

c) Unsatisfactory specimens must be reported to the section supervisor within 15 minutes of receiving them.

5 10% PREPARE SPECIMENS FOR REFERENCE LABS AND COMPLETE REQUEST FORMS

a) There must be no more than three specimens per year sent to the wrong reference lab.

b) There must be no more than one specimen per month not properly prepared or with an incomplete work request.

c) There must be no more than one specimen per month not ready for pickup at the scheduled time.

C. Section maintenance (10%)

6 2% STOCK EARLY MORNING COLLECTION BASKETS

a) Supplies in the basket must be adequate to meet collection needs.

7 2% MAINTAIN APPEARANCE OF BLOOD COLLECTION AREA

a) Must clean countertops daily.

b) Must stock supplies neatly.

c) Overall appearance must be regarded as satisfactory by the supervisor.

8 5% MAINTAIN INVENTORY OF SUPPLIES

a) The supervisor must be notified of weekly needs by Friday.

b) Problems or backorders must be promptly reported to the supervisors.

9	**1%**	**PROVIDE SUPERVISOR WITH TOTAL NEEDLE AND LANCET COUNT**

a) Must provide an accurate count by the fifth working day of each month.

D. Miscellaneous (5%)

10	**3%**	**UPDATE ROLODEX AND BLOOD COLLECTION MANUAL**

a) These records must be updated within one week after changes are initiated.

b) Rolodex and manual must be reviewed annually.

11	**2%**	**TRAIN NEW EMPLOYEES AND STUDENTS**

a) The evaluation of the trainee must be submitted to the supervisor within 48 hours after completing the training.

b) Employee and student feedback (orientation questionnaire) must indicate satisfactory training.

c) There must be no more than two discrepancies per year between stated policy and actual training, as noted by the supervisor.

E. Special

12	**—**	**MAINTAIN PERSONAL APPEARANCE**

a) There must be no more than three violations of appearance code per year.

13	**—**	**MAINTAIN COOPERATIVE ATTITUDE WITH LABORATORY STAFF**

a) There must be no more than three valid complaints per year from staff members.

Position description—Clinical laboratory

Title: Secretary/Receptionist   **Section:** Laboratory office
Shift: Evening and weekend   **Pay grade:** 040
Prepared by: S. Yohe

Functions:

Process laboratory reports.

Answer laboratory phones.

Prepare necessary forms for donors and outpatients.

Qualifications:

High school graduate.

General typing skills.

Reports to:

Administrative assistant.

Supervises:

No one.

Coordinates with:

Evening and weekend lab supervisors.

Floor nurses.

Limits of authority   **Class**

1. Organize own workload, setting priorities, speed, etc.   1

2. On incoming calls, decide whether to transfer the call or
   handle it.   1

A. Laboratory reports (50%)

1 25% PROCESS INPATIENT AND OUTPATIENT REPORTS

a) The originals of inpatient reports must be time-stamped and sent or delivered to nursing stations at the times established in the laboratory service manual.

b) The originals of outpatient reports must be correctly placed in physicians' folders or boxes or mailed.

c) File copies must be filed (if properly authorized) or saved for the day supervisor's signature if required.

d) Charge slips must be correctly batched and delivered to the data processing department by the end of the shift.

2 5% PROCESS REPORTS FROM REFERENCE LABORATORIES

a) Reference lab reports must be correctly matched with our request form.

b) The reports must be stamped with the pathologist's name and placed in his "in" box by 10:30 a.m.

3 5% PREPARE LAB SLIPS FOR SPECIMENS DELIVERED DIRECTLY TO THE LAB

a) Request forms must be correctly prepared, time-stamped, and delivered to the blood collection section within 30 minutes of receiving the specimen.

4 15% MAINTAIN LABORATORY FILES

a) Must complete filing left from the day shift.

b) Misfiling must be no greater than others working the main desk.

123

B. Telephone (35%)

5 30% HANDLE INCOMING PHONE CALLS

a) Must answer questions or report test results within 60 seconds.

b) Must route calls to the correct section or individual requested without disconnecting the call.

c) Must operate both types of phones in the lab.

6 5% CALL STAT OR TO-BE-CALLED REPORTS

a) Calls must be made within five minutes of receiving the report.

C. Miscellaneous (15%)

7 10% PROCESS BLOOD DONOR FORMS

a) The donor must be taken care of within two minutes of arriving.

b) Forms must be correctly prepared within 10 minutes.

c) Must instruct the donor to answer questions, sign the form, and send him to the blood bank.

d) There must be no more than one valid complaint per year from donors regarding poor service.

8 5% PREPARE ENVELOPES FOR PHYSICIAN MAILING AND BLANK CORONARY FORMS

a) Envelopes must be available for all physicians having reports mailed out.

b) Blank coronary requisition forms including hematology, biochemistry, and two liver/lipid request forms must be available on all three shifts.

9 — MAINTAIN ATTITUDE AND MORALE (SEE PAGES 98-103)

Position description—Clinical laboratory

Title: Medical technician   **Section:** Chemistry

Shift: First   **Pay grade:** 080   **Prepared by:** S. Yohe

Functions:

Perform routine chemistry and urinalysis procedures.

Qualifications:

CLA (ASCP), MLT (ASCP), or equivalent.

Reports to:

Chemistry bench supervisor.

Supervises:

No one.

Coordinates with:

Other section personnel.

Limits of authority	Class
1. Perform repeat tests when results are questionable.	2
2. Judge the adequacy of submitted specimens. Request an additional specimen if unsatisfactory.	1

A. Chemistry tests (95%)

1 | 85%   **PERFORM TESTS ON CHEMISTRY AND URINALYSIS PROCEDURE LIST**

a) Must learn new procedures added to the test list.

b) Procedures must be performed within the stated turnaround time at least 90 percent of the time.

c) There must be no more than three complaints (incident reports) per year from physicians or nursing personnel regarding personally performed procedures.

2 | 4%   **TRANSCRIBE TEST RESULTS ON REPORT FORMS**

a) The report must include initials of technician.

b) Results must be legible and neat.

c) The report must include information regarding abnormal appearance of specimen or be marked satisfactory.

d) Abnormal results must be circled.

3 | 1%   **REPORT PANIC OR TO-BE-CALLED VALUES BY TELEPHONE**

a) These results must be called within 15 minutes of completing the test.

b) The report must document that the result was called and the time of the call.

4 | 5%   **PERFORM DESIGNATED QC PROCEDURES**

a) There must be no more than two valid complaints per year from the supervisor.

b) Must sign log books when performing QC procedures at least 90 percent of time.

c) Must report corrective action for QC problems on KDA at least 90 percent of time.

5 | — | **NOTIFY BENCH SUPERVISOR WHEN SUPPLIES, TEST KITS, OR REAGENTS SHOULD BE REORDERED**

a) There must be no more than two lapses per year.

B. Miscellaneous (5%)

6 | 5% | **PERFORM BLOOD COLLECTION PROCEDURES**

a) There must be no more than one complaint per year from nurses, physicians, or the phlebotomy supervisor concerning method of blood collection, attitude, or courtesy.

7 | — | **MAINTAIN ATTITUDE AND MORALE**

a) There must be no more than one valid complaint per year from other lab personnel regarding cooperation.

b) There must be no more than one safety violation per year.

c) Annual sick time must be equal to or better than laboratory average.

d) Must return from lunch and breaks promptly.

e) Must report to work on time 95 percent of the time.

f) Must remain after hours at the request of the technical supervisor to complete work, 80 percent of the time requested.

8 | — | **MAINTAIN ATTITUDE AND MORALE (SEE PAGES 98-103)**

Position description—Clinical laboratory

Title: Medical technician   **Section:** Hematology
Shift: First   **Pay grade:** 080   **Prepared by:** S. Yohe

Functions:
Perform routine hematology and coagulation procedures.

Qualifications:
CLA (ASCP), MLT (ASCP), or equivalent.

Reports to:
Hematology bench supervisor.

Supervises:
No one.

Coordinates with:
Other section personnel.

Limits of authority	Class
1. Perform repeat tests when results are questionable.	2
2. Judge the adequacy of submitted specimens. Request an additional specimen if unsatisfactory.	1

A. Hematology and coagulation procedures (95%)

1 | 85% | PERFORM ROUTINE HEMATOLOGY AND COAGULATION PROCEDURES AS LISTED IN THE LABORATORY SERVICE MANUAL

a) Daily PT, PTTs and CBCs without differentials must be reported by 9:30 a.m. 80 percent of the time.

b) CBCs with differentials must be reported by 1:30 a.m. at least 85 percent of the time.

c) All Stat procedures must be performed within limits of turnaround times.

d) No more than 5 percent of differentials reviewed by the supervisor shall be rated as unsatisfactory or poor.

2 | 4% | REPORT RESULTS OF HEMATOLOGY AND COAGULATION PROCEDURES

a) Abnormal results must be circled.

b) Slips must be neat, legible, dated, and initialed when submitted to the supervisor.

c) There must be no more than two clerical errors per month, as noted by the supervisor.

d) There must be no more than two documented complaints per year involving reported patient results.

3 | 1% | SPECIAL HANDLING OF REPORTS

a) Panic values and to-be-called results must be called within 15 minutes of completing the test.

b) Time of call must be documented on the lab request.

4 | 5% | PERFORM DESIGNATED QC PROCEDURES

a) There must be no more than two complaints per month from the supervisor for failure to document daily QC.

129

b) Results that do not correlate must be identified and reported to the supervisor.

c) The supervisor must be notified at least 90 percent of the time if QC results are out of the established range.

B. Miscellaneous (5%)

5 3% PROVIDE ASSISTANCE IN BLOOD COLLECTION

a) Must be available to collect blood upon request by the blood collection supervisor.

b) There must be no more than two valid complaints per year from patients regarding technique.

c) Must not perform more than two venipunctures on the same patient.

d) There must be no more than two complaints per year from physicians or nurses regarding improper blood collection.

6 2% PURSUE A CONTINUING EDUCATION PROGRAM

a) Must meet the minimum requirements for CE units.

7 — MAINTAIN ATTITUDE AND MORALE

a) There must be no more than one valid complaint per year from other lab personnel regarding cooperation.

b) There must be no more than one safety violation per year.

c) Annual sick time must be equal to or better than the laboratory average.

d) Must return from lunch and breaks promptly.

e) Must report to work on time 95 percent of the time.

f) Must remain after hours at the request of the bench supervisor to complete work.

Position description—Clinical laboratory

Title: Medical technician   **Section:** General
Shift: Second   **Pay grade:** 080   **Prepared by:** S. Yohe

Functions:

Perform and interpret routine diagnostic procedures in chemistry, hematology, microbiology, and immunohematology.

Qualifications:

CLA(ASCP), MLT(ASCP), or equivalent.

Reports to:

Evening supervisor.

Supervises:

No one.

Coordinates with:

Shift personnel, hospital evening administrator.

Limits of authority	Class
1. Perform repeat tests when results are questionable.	2
2. Judge the adequacy of submitted specimens and request another specimen if necessary.	1
3. Modify work patterns to facilitate daily workload.	1
4. Assign Stat test priorities.	1
5. Give telephone reports when requested by authorized personnel, and call physicians or nurses with panic values.	1

A. Technical procedures (80%)

1 | 20% **PERFORM TESTS ON CHEMISTRY AND URINALYSIS PROCEDURE LIST**

a) Procedures must be performed within the stated turnaround time at least 90 percent of the time.

b) Must learn new procedures added to the test list.

c) Analyze QC data for each procedure, record values on appropriate log sheets, and report to supervisor when results are outside two standard deviations.

d) There must be no more than three complaints (incident reports) per year from physicians or nursing personnel regarding personally performed procedures.

2 | 20% **PERFORM TESTS ON HEMATOLOGY AND COAGULATION PROCEDURE LIST**

a) Procedures must be performed within the stated turnaround time at least 90 percent of the time.

b) Must learn new procedures added to the test list.

c) No more than 5 percent of differentials reviewed by supervisor shall be rated as unsatisfactory or poor.

3 | 20% **PERFORM ROUTINE BACTERIOLOGY PRO- CEDURES INCLUDING READING OF PLATES, IDENTIFICATION, AND ANTIBIOTIC SUSCEPTI- BILITY TESTING OF SUSPECTED PATHOGENS**

a) Cultures must be planted on appropriate media within 15 minutes.

b) Stat Gram stains must be prepared or interpreted within 30 minutes of receiving the specimen.

c) Must read plates and set up necessary tests by 10:00 p.m.

d) All procedures must be performed according to laboratory specifications.

4 15% PERFORM ROUTINE TESTS ON IMMUNO-HEMATOLOGY STAT PROCEDURE LIST

a) Procedures must be performed within the stated turnaround time at least 90 percent of the time.

b) Blood availability or compatibility problems must be immediately reported to the supervisor or pathologist on call.

5 5% ISSUE BLOOD AND PREPARE COMPONENTS LISTED IN THE BLOOD BANK TRANSFUSION MANUAL

a) All blood and components must be prepared according to AABB and FDA standards.

B. Report results—all sections (10%)

6 5% TRANSCRIBE TEST RESULTS ON REPORT FORMS

a) The report must include initials of technologist.

b) Results must be legible and neat.

c) The report must include information regarding abnormal appearance of specimen or be marked satisfactory.

d) Abnormal results must be circled.

7 5% SPECIAL HANDLING OF REPORTS

a) Panic values and to-be-called results must be called within 15 minutes of completing the test.

b) Time of call must be documented on lab request.

133

C. Miscellaneous (10%)

8 | 10% | COLLECT BLOOD SPECIMENS FROM HOSPITAL INPATIENTS AND OUTPATIENTS

a) Stats and timed requests must be done within 10 minutes.

b) Multiple venipuncture rate must not be higher than 5 percent of total venipunctures.

c) Unsuccessful venipunctures must not be higher than 5 percent of total venipunctures.

9 | — | MAINTAIN ATTITUDE AND MORALE

a) There must be no more than one valid complaint per year from other lab personnel regarding cooperation.

b) There must be no more than one safety violation per year.

c) Annual sick time must be equal to or better than the laboratory average.

d) Must return from dinner within 30 minutes and from breaks within 20 minutes.

e) Must report to work on time 95 percent of the time.

f) Must remain after hours at the request of the supervisor to complete work.

Position description—Clinical laboratory

Title: Medical technician **Section:** Microbiology
Shift: First **Pay grade:** 080 **Prepared by:** W. George

Functions:
Perform routine microbiology and serology procedures.

Qualifications:
CLA (ASCP), MLT (ASCP), or equivalent.

Reports to:
Microbiology bench supervisor.

Supervises:
No one.

Coordinates with:
Other section personnel.

Limits of authority	Class
1. Perform repeat tests when results are questionable.	2
2. Judge the adequacy of submitted specimens. Request an additional specimen if unsatisfactory.	1
3. Organize daily work.	1

A. Microbiology tests (65%)

1	50%

PERFORM ROUTINE BACTERIOLOGY PRO-CEDURES INCLUDING READING OF PLATES, IDENTIFICATION, AND ANTIBIOTIC SUSCEPTI-BILITY TESTING OF SUSPECTED PATHOGENS

a) Cultures must be planted on appropriate media within 15 minutes.

b) Stat Gram stains must be prepared and stained within 15 minutes of specimen receipt; a technologist must interpret them.

c) Must read plates and set up routine tests by 3 p.m.

d) Must consult with a technologist on unusual isolates.

e) All procedures must be performed according to laboratory specifications.

f) Must recognize and report unusual final results to supervisor.

g) There must be no more than three complaints (incident reports) per year from physicians or nursing personnel regarding bacteriology results and procedures.

2	5%

PERFORM ROUTINE AFB WORK INCLUDING SPECIMEN PROCESSING AND STAINING

a) Smears of specimens must be processed, cultured, and prepared within one hour.

b) Must read stains within 15 minutes and notify the supervisor if a result is questionable or positive.

c) All procedures must be performed according to laboratory specifications.

3	2%

PERFORM ROUTINE MYCOLOGY INCLUDING SPECIMEN PLANTING AND VARIOUS STAINING PROCEDURES

a) Smears of specimens must be planted and prepared within 15 minutes.

b) Must perform and read Gram stains, India ink, and KOH preparations within 30 minutes and notify supervisor if results are questionable or positive.

c) All procedures must be performed according to laboratory specifications.

4   4%   PERFORM ROUTINE PARASITOLOGY WORK INCLUDING SPECIMEN PROCESSING, STAINING PROCEDURES, AND PARASITE IDENTIFICATION

a) Specimens must be examined and placed in preservatives within 10 minutes.

b) Must prepare and read direct smears and stained smears within two hours and notify supervisor if results are questionable or positive.

c) Fecal specimens must be concentrated within one hour.

d) All procedures must be performed according to laboratory specifications.

5   2%   REPORT RESULTS

a) Written reports must be legible, neat, and accurate 85 percent of the time.

b) Report must include date, technician's initials, and time the specimen was planted or processed.

c) Stat reports, positive blood and CSF cultures, and other necessary results must be called, noted on the report form, and brought to the attention of the supervisor.

6   2%   PERFORM MICROBIOLOGY QUALITY CONTROL

a) There must be no more than one complaint per year.

(1)	(2)	Duty/Performance Standards
		b) QC results must be recorded on appropriate sheets, dated, and initialed.
		c) Must notify supervisor of out-of-control results.

B. Serology tests (25%)

7	22%	**PERFORM ROUTINE AND SPECIAL SEROLOGY PROCEDURES**

a) All procedures must be performed within stated turnaround times at least 85 percent of the time.

b) Must learn new procedures as added.

c) Abnormal and unusual results must be recognized and reported to the supervisor.

d) There must be no more than three complaints per year from physicians or nursing personnel regarding serology results and procedures.

e) All procedures must be performed according to laboratory specifications.

8	2%	**REPORT RESULTS**

a) Written reports must be legible, neat, and accurate 85 percent of the time.

b) The report must state whether the specimen is satisfactory or unsatisfactory, and be dated and initialed.

c) Stat, to-be-called, and other necessary results must be called and noted on the report form.

9	1%	**PERFORM SEROLOGY QUALITY CONTROL**

a) There must be no more than one complaint per year.

b) QC results must be recorded on appropriate sheets, dated, and initialed.

c) Must notify supervisor of out-of-control results.

(1)	(2)	

C. Skin tests (2%)

10 **2%** **ADMINISTER INTRACUTANEOUS SKIN TESTS**

a) Must inject each skin test within 10 minutes.

b) Test must be given in accordance with standard procedure.

c) There must be no more than one complaint per year from physicians or nursing personnel regarding administration of skin tests.

D. Miscellaneous (18%)

11 **6%** **MEDIA AND REAGENTS**

a) Must prepare required media and reagents as requested by supervisor.

12 **2%** **ACHIEVE AT LEAST THE MINIMUM CONTINU-ING EDUCATION CREDITS**

a) Must attend at least 50 percent of laboratory staff and section meetings.

b) Must attend required hospital meetings.

13 **—** **MAINTAIN ATTITUDE AND MORALE**

a) There must be no more than one valid complaint per year from other laboratory personnel regarding cooperation.

b) There must be no more than one safety violation per year.

c) Annual sick time must be equal to or better than the laboratory average.

d) Must return from lunch and breaks promptly.

e) Must report to work on time 95 percent of the time.

f) Must remain after hours at the request of the technical supervisor to complete work 80 percent of the time requested.

Index

*Italic page numbers refer to tables
and figures.

Other Titles of Related Interest From
Medical Economics Books

Interviewing Skills for Laboratory Supervisors
By William O. Umiker, M.D.
ISBN 0-87489-367-4

The Effective Laboratory Supervisor
By William O. Umiker, M.D.
ISBN 0-87489-269-4

Clinical Decision Levels for Lab Tests
Bernard E. Statland, M.D., Ph.D.
ISBN 0-87489-301-1

Legal Guidelines for the Clinical Laboratory
Edited by Robert J. Fitzgibbon
ISBN 0-87489-243-0

*A Practical Guide to Financial Management of
the Clinical Laboratory*
By Janiece Sattler
ISBN 0-87489-235-X

Sharpening Laboratory Management Skills
Compiled and edited by Edward M. Friedman
ISBN 0-87489-204-X

Managing the Patient-Focused Laboratory
By George D. Lundberg, M.D.
ISBN 0-87489-065-9

*Laboratory Diagnosis and Patient Monitoring:
Clinical Chemistry*
Edited by Robert S. Galen, M.D., and Leslie Brennan
ISBN 0-87489-265-1

For information, write to:
Customer Service Manager
Medical Economics Books
Oradell, NJ 07649

Or dial toll-free: 1-800-223-0581, ext. 2755
(Within the 201 area: 262-3030, ext. 2755)